FACING the REALITY

Based on the true story of one woman's journey
to find love in the age of HIV/AIDS

by C.J. Greene

authorHOUSE®

AuthorHouse™
1663 Liberty Drive
Bloomington, IN 47403
www.authorhouse.com
Phone: 1 (800) 839-8640

Published by AuthorHouse 03/18/2020

ISBN: 978-1-4343-7731-9 (sc)

Print information available on the last page.

ACKNOWLEDGEMENTS

This book is dedicated to my children,

and my family...

to whom I give all of my love.

I am truly sorry if I have ever given you any grief in this life, believe me, ... that was not my intention.

Sometimes, you just can't see the forest for all of the trees.

CONTENTS

Facing the Reality

is based on a true story.

The characters in this book are fictional.

Any resemblance to persons living or dead is

purely coincidental, and are mere

characterizations for fictional content only.

PREFACE

From the Star Nation Prophesy

COPYRIGHT © Wolf Lodge 1997

TRUTH OR CONSEQUENCES

This is a very different time, unlike any time that has ever existed on this plane before. For most of you, there is the tendency to see nothing, no future and no past. As a result, many see this time we are living in now as a time of confusion and suffering, a time of hopelessness. But this is not the essence of this time, nor is it the purpose of this experience.

May the people of the Earth hear this message of information and hope. May they again reach inside and touch the love that has always been there for them from the union of the Father and the Mother To the undiscerning mind, this can be seen as a time of the greatest conflict that ever existed within the souls of mankind.

We would ask you then to consider:

Where is your heart commitment?

What does your inner guidance tell you?

You must believe in yourself, in your own Divinity. If you do not believe in yourself, how can you put faith in the concept that some Heavenly Host would even consider taking you up in a great ship or through the experience of Divine Rapture? These are children's fairy tales, created to manufacture false hope in the hopeless.

We bid you farewell. Go forth with love; know that you are the Children of the Sun.

INTRODUCTION

THERE IS NO SUCH THING AS A COINCIDENCE

It's Just God's Way of Remaining Anonymous

"The Lord works in mysterious ways…" is something we have all heard at one time or another. But, it never ceases to amaze me when he shows his handiworks in our lives as an affirmation of his existence. Sometimes we all need a reminder every now and then, that the Lord is alive and well, and living inside of us all when we finally do acknowledge his existence.

The burdens of my current life weighed heavily on my mind, as I rode to the meeting of the Sister's Circle with my sister-in-law, early last September. She is an evangelist, and I had become accustomed to talking to her about my family and personal problems. It was comforting to know that there was someone out there willing to listen to the ramblings of a middle-aged, overworked, under-appreciated, single mother.

She too, had been a single parent at one time and I knew that she would understand my angst. But, to tell the truth, I envied her seemingly perfect married life. I wanted to find out **HER SECRET** to happiness.

She was well aware of our family problems; having spoken about them to my brother, and she later told me that they had prayed together that a breakthrough miracle might happen to quell the tensions in our family. I had just begun staying with them for the few days that it would take me to make a dress for her. Thus, I got the chance to observe her daily routine on a more intimate basis.

This was a unique arrangement for us because usually she would come to my house on Long Island for her fittings, etc., but this time we felt that it might be better for me to come and stay with her for the duration of the construction of her dress. I worried about my thirteen year old son back home on Long Island, and whether or not the house would run smoothly without my nagging presence, so I wanted to get the job finished as soon as possible.

BUT, IT SEEMS THE LORD HAD OTHER PLANS FOR ME!

I was thinking about my money problems, and worrying about how I was going to pay an old bill that would allow me to get a new apartment, and clear up my credit report,--- but, I really didn't want to talk about that. I was about to tell her about something else that was truly disturbing me. I am a normally talkative person, so as we rode through New York City, naturally, I struck up a conversation. It was about a twenty or thirty minute ride from her house in New York to the meeting place in New Jersey, so we had ample time to kill.

At first we were talking about survival issues, and about how she had received a small pamphlet from some people who were handing them out on the street because of the obvious concerns with the coming of the anniversary of the September 11th terrorist attacks that coming Monday. I asked her a question about **"The Last Days"** and what her beliefs were on the subject.

We spoke briefly about my own religious beliefs, which I had explained to her were **"NEW AGE"**, and that I was a believing, but non-practicing Buddhist; and that I did not put a name on the Universal power that I believed controlled our lives. I told her that I merely waited for that power to show itself to me, and that I used it to guide me in my life.

Our conversation somehow turned to what the attitude of young people is about sex these days, and about how **God had sent the plagues of AIDS, HIV,** and the myriad of other venereal and sexually transmitted diseases down on to the earth to show us how the sins of illicit, promiscuous, sex and the controversy behind homosexuality can destroy people's lives. I grew up in the middle of the so-called Sexual Revolution of the 1970's, and I am well aware of the evolution of people's sexual morals leading to the horrible death and destruction that AIDS has caused in our world today.

I've written this novel about it, and have lost several friends and relatives to the disease. This led me to reveal to her the real issue that had been weighing on my mind; that of whether or not I should move back to Atlanta, Georgia where I had met a man five years previously with whom I had been having a sexual relationship. And, to illustrate the urgency of my problem, I was supposed to have been moving within a week, right after I finished her dress.

I will remind you that I am a fifty-two year old woman, so I should really know about the dangers of premarital sex and/or relationships based solely on sex. But, I began telling her about my **"obsession"** and about how people did not understand the true meaning of the word. An obsession is a lot like an addiction, like an addiction to drugs like Crack, Ecstasy, or Heroin. It is an uncontrollable (?) urge to do something, to have something, or to be with someone.

I began explaining to her about my attraction for this man, whom after much introspection, I came realize, was just using me for sex. But, I could not see it that way at first because in my mind, I was desperate for the little bit of attention that he gave to me when we were together while I was going through the pain of losing my mother. He was the only man with whom I had been having sex in over two years.

It was not like I did not have other friends, or that he was so unusually attractive, or that he had spent a lot of money on me, or even that he had treated me particularly nice, --- it was mainly the feelings I got from chasing the illusive "high" that I achieved from having sex with him. Then, I described to her that long dark, endless tunnel that perversion and sin leads you down, sucks you into, drains you of your energy, and the horrendous pain that you experience trying to get out of that tunnel. I knew that I did not want to experience that ever again in my life, as I had been there (done that) in the days of my naïve youth.

I had not heard from the man in a while, since I had moved back to New York, and after calling him practically every day for a month and leaving multiple messages; begging him to tell me what was going on in his head and in his life, before I moved back to Atlanta. So, I called him the night before and he finally answered the phone. But, he didn't answer it to actually talk to me, he merely clicked on the phone to let me hear him having sex with another woman!

But, I didn't get enraged or jealous in the normal sense of the word as you might think I would have, because I knew that neither of us was being exclusive. I was so angry that he had chosen to throw it in my face (so to speak) instead of talking to me about it. I left him several nasty messages, and the next day, to satisfy my growing disdain of his behavior, I called him again, to see if he would talk to me about what he had done the night before.

This time, he actually answered the phone and told me in no uncertain terms, that if I came back to Atlanta and called to see him, again, that I would have to be willing to engage in multiple sex partner activities, threesomes, homosexual acts, etc., or else he would not see me. This was a new development for us...but, what we *didn't know* was that...

GOD HAD OTHER PLANS FOR ME.

My sister-in-law and I rode on to the meeting still discussing my problems. I did not know what to expect when we arrived, and I tried to quell my apprehension at meeting new people in an unfamiliar place. I am a normally friendly person, but I am unusually quiet and shy when I don't know where I am going or what I will be doing when I get there. Most people think that I am standoffish or stuck up when I don't interact with them right away, so I was trying my best to "fit in" this time. So, I gravitated to the front where Sister Marlene, the prayer leader, was sitting reading her Bible. I struck up a conversation with her.

She had been reading a passage in Corinthians, about **GOD SHOWING US HIS POWER,** and I began to feel more comfortable.

Another sister came in and introduced herself to me. Her name was Ruth, and I told her that my mother's name was also Ruth, (and anyone who is familiar with the Masons will know that Ruth was the

Gleaner in the Bible, and that it was also my station in the lodge when I was a Eastern Star.) I began to feel much, much better. Sister Janet introduced herself to me and mentioned that I looked familiar to her. (Little did she know that she favored my own sister). I observed; trying hard to not get lost in the newspaper in which I was reading an article about of all things **"SEXUAL ADDICTIONS."**

I couldn't help but notice how much Sister Marlene bore a striking resemblance to my deceased mother, who had just recently passed away, and whom I was missing terribly. Another sister reminded me of my niece. Another reminded me of a friend that I had in college. I started feeling even more comfortable.

Then, Sister Gwen told her hilarious story about getting her car fixed, and how she needed nearly $4000 which she didn't have to pay the bill. She spoke about how she hesitated to ask her soon-to-be ex-husband for the money; for fear of being obligated to repay someone she was trying to get out of her life. She told us how **GOD MADE A WAY OUT OF NO WAY** for her.

Then, Sister Marcia, told her story of getting arrested at a most inconvenient time, but she managed to "beat the charge" because her friend worked for the Sheriff's Dept., and was the one who **HANDLED THE PROBLEM FOR HER**. But it was really **GOD**, not her friend, who had **MADE A WAY OUT OF NO WAY** for her. They showed us that we do not need to rely on friends, family, lovers, or strangers to get us out of trouble, and that all we need is the **POWER OF THE LORD** to make a way for us.

Then, Sister Janet gave her speech about the seven **"essions"** that hold us back from God's Glory: **Regression, Repression, Oppression, Suppression, Depression, OBSESSION, and Possession.** I immediately began to think: **"Now I know why I came here tonight...This message was for me."**

When my beautiful sister-in-law told everyone that I was making a dress for her, when The Lord instructed her to stop my worldly work, so that I could come and see his work being done, that was when I knew that:

GOD HAD OTHER PLANS FOR ME.

I decided to let HIM tell me where he wants me to live, and what HE wants me to do, and to not worry about how it was going to get done. The sisters of this congregation showed me the love that no trifling, sex-obsessed, human being could ever show me. They showed me that when we are patient and wait on the Lord-- that **A WAY CAN BE MADE OUT OF NO WAY.**

Although I am a three-times baptized, born again, holy sanctified, re-affirmed, non-practicing, self-made Buddhist/Kemetic Christian...

I ACCEPTED THE NAME OF THE LORD JESUS CHRIST BACK INTO MY LIFE THAT NIGHT and rededicated my life to doing HIS WORK.

However, when you make a promise to yourself, and especially when you make a promise to God, you had better follow through, or else you may have to deal with some very nasty consequences for your actions. And if you don't believe me, listen to what happened to me...

Three months later, I had moved back to Atlanta, and was living with an old friend of mine in her lovely home on the outskirts of the city. The temptation was tremendous for me to call my old sex partner, and I fought the desire to do so...for about three days. It was difficult for me to get out of my friend's house late at night, because she would come home from work at about 7 PM and, promptly at 9 PM she would put the house on "lock down," turn on the alarms, and go to bed. The only way in or out of the house was through her garage, which was right below her bedroom, so sneaking out in the middle of the night would have been nearly impossible.

I felt like a teenager locked in their parent's home, or a prisoner in the county jail. She was a very staunch Christian, and I wasn't about to disrespect her home. So, I decided that I needed a plan. I was going to *lie to her* instead. I told my friend that I was going to visit my niece, in another part of town, and that I would be spending the night at her house.

The plan worked like a charm, and I ended up going to see my old sex buddy for a night of fun and games. Sure, I felt a little guilty about telling her the lie, but the feeling that I got when I was with him, made up for all the bad feelings I'd had, and we picked up right where we had left off ten months ago. I had only seen him that one time when something very unexpected happened to me.

I, suddenly, started having problems on my temporary job and got unceremoniously, dropped from the agency I was working for, therefore I had no money to buy presents or to take care of myself or my family at the worst time of the year...the Christmas holidays! Two weeks later, my ex-husband decided to not pay his child support that month and then, my friend and I had a disagreement one night,...not about money....but, about something entirely unrelated to my living in her home.

She claimed that it had nothing to do with my financial situation, but I felt uncomfortable living with her any longer. I decided that I was going to move out and go stay with my niece, who owed me some money.

Unfortunately, my niece suffered from a very serious bi-polar disorder, had had a nasty psychotic episode prior to my moving in with her, and I ended up sleeping in my car at the worst time of the year in near zero degree weather.

Ironically, the man with whom I had been having sex for almost three years, and with whom I had had sex <u>the very night</u> that I moved out of my friend's house, told me that I could not stay with him, and although he was living in a very nice FOUR BEDROOM HOUSE all by himself, that he did not want any roommates...especially not a woman who might cramp his style; not even for a few weeks. The morning I left his house it was raining cats and dogs; a cold and nasty kind of February rain. I had nowhere else to go.

To make matters worse, my cell phone got cut off, and I had no way to communicate with employers or my family who, curiously, at the worse time of my life, also decided that they were not going to help me get into a safe, warm place to live ---so, I ended up going to a Salvation Army shelter in the city for assistance.

While I was at the shelter, I met a very nice woman who introduced me to a man who was an old friend of hers, and within a few days, I had gone to go live with them in the man's apartment, since the shelter was a very noisy, inconvenient, and unfriendly place to live, for the most part. The arrangement worked out, perfectly, and luckily, since I was expecting some Student Loan funds to come through along with my Income Tax Refund, within about a week I had moved into a luxury apartment owned by the school I was attending and started sharing it with some other students. It wasn't my own, but it was a safe, warm, quiet and clean place to stay while I continued my studies.

All this sounds really good doesn't it? I felt blessed and loved. The only problem was that, although they were very nice, and I had a very enlightening and spiritual experience living with them, the two people that I had befriended turned out to be Crack heads! They had carefully hid their addictions from me, but soon, they were sneaking out to go buy their drugs in the middle of the night, and asking me for money to support their habits. When I moved out, I decided that I couldn't associate with them any longer. So then, I had lost the only friends I had there, and started feeling very lonely again, indeed.

However, while I was staying at the shelter I had also met someone else. I became attracted to a man who worked his spiritual magic on me, told me everything I wanted and needed to hear, vowed undying love for me, and almost moved into my student apartment with me. We started having sex on a regular basis and planning a life together. Unfortunately, he was already married, separated from his wife, and could only plan but so much of a life with me, until he could get a divorce from her. (Can you say: "Adulterer"?) To make matters worse, I was still seeing my previous sex partner (Yes, the one who refused to take me in) on the side. I was bouncing between these two men like a tennis ball at Wimbledon; having the time of my life. That is...Until the S**t Hit the Fan.

Now...I know you have a lot of questions at this point.

1. How could I possibly start a "relationship" with a married man, especially one who was living in a shelter; someone who I didn't really know from Adam? Well...I'll tell you...he was good--- just too good to be true. Like I said--- He talked a good game. He told me what I wanted to hear, and made promises that he couldn't keep. We got along extremely well together, and he was very good company when there was no one else around. He appealed to my martyr-motherly side, and played on my good graces.

He told me he loved me, (something the other man had never done) and besides that,...the sex with him was mind boggling! He knew all the right moves and all the things to do to make a woman feel special. My relation-ship with him actually made my relationship with the other man, (that is if you want to call what we had a "relationship") even better.

Somehow, the other man found out about him, so then he viewed the situation as a competition to prove that he was the better man in bed. Then, I got greedy and started heading straight for that slippery slope to Hell, known as **OBSESSION.** I had already become a liar and an Adulteress; in what other perversions could I possibly indulge?

And, I know you have a lot of other questions to ask me right about now:

2. Did we use protection? Of course, we did, that is... until the condom broke! (Well now, that put a big damper on the fun and games, didn't it?) As a matter of fact, the day that the condom broke, I went from having sex with one man, right to having sex with the other man, (the one with whom I had *never* used a condom) that same night. We figured that since the condom had broke and he knew that he was clean, that we might as well forget about using a condom any more. He just wanted an excuse to not use one in the first place and I couldn't ask my first friend to suddenly start using a condom, because then he would start asking questions that I didn't want to answer at that point. That was when I was about to get sucked into the middle of one the deepest **OBSESSIONS** I had ever experienced in my entire life

3. Why would I want to have anything to do with a man who had virtually kicked me into the streets in a freezing rain to be homeless? That is what **OBSESSION** does to you. It robs you of your dignity, self-esteem and everything else that is important to you. You do not think rationally, and you no longer care what happens to you, --- all you care about it whether or not you can be with or have the object of your desire. Again, I was chasing that "high" that came from having sex with him, in order to anesthetize my feelings and take my mind off my problems. I was hooked on my own orgasms.

4. Why didn't my religious beliefs stop me from doing this? Because everyone else was doing it, too! We all know that people who go to church are some of the biggest hypocrites on earth. I am quite sure you know a bunch of people who go to church *every* Sunday, and they are all smoking, drinking, lying, having premarital sex, taking drugs, being angry and envious...*whatever*, ... every other day of the week.

Going to church does not make you stop sinning.

People go to church to ask God for *forgiveness* from their sins, right? I went to church with my "crack head" friends all the time. They were the first ones to jump up and yell: "Hallelujah!" when the preacher started talking about deliverance.

Only the realization that **YOU WILL BE PUNISHED** for your wrong actions and **KARMA** is the **ONLY THING** that will stop you from continuing an **OBSESSION OR ADDICTION.**

5. What happened after we stopped using the condoms? Well...after a big argument about not being sincere in his motives for being with me, the man I had met at the shelter, finally gave me the proof that he really was HIV negative. (Whew!) But then, I had to tell my other sex partner that he needed to get tested to make sure he was alright, and I also had to tell him that I wasn't having sex with the guy from the shelter, anymore. He cursed me out, told me that I was a nasty whore, refused to see me anymore, and then he decided that he was going to treat me even more badly than he was already treating me by not talking to me.

Yes, the guy from the shelter was HIV negative **BUT**...and this is a big one...**HE WAS A SYPHILLIS CARRIER!** So, now I may have been infected with a very serious venereal disease that can lay dormant in your body for ten years or more! Not only that...I may have infected my other sex partner, too. Today, neither one of the men are in my life, and I am alone again...to ponder my fate.

6. Why did I do this to myself? I ask myself this question every day. And, the only thing I can say is this: I was a very lonely, frustrated, old lady, looking for love in all the wrong places, too gullible, too stupid, and too greedy to know what was good for me. I am only human. **And, there is NO FOOL LIKE AN OLD FOOL.**

But seriously, I was sexually molested several times between the ages of 10 and 14, and I had never told anyone in my family about this. My knowledge about sex and how to relate to men in healthy ways was definitely severely damaged at a very early age. Add to that the fact that I did not grow up with a strong male father figure in my life, and you get a pretty messed up adult. To think I needed to go through this in order to let other people see how easy it is to slip up on the way to Righteousness...right in the face of an **OBSESSION.**

So now... you can decide for yourself exactly what you need to do to stop *yourself* from making the same mistakes. Do not judge me because it is not your place to judge. Everything happens for a reason and you are never too old (and sometimes, not too young) to learn. Hopefully, you will read my story and learn something very valuable. It is based on my life, although it is totally fiction. I wrote it to make a very serious point...

All the religion in the world cannot save you from sinning if you yourself are not strong enough to overcome your sin.

Religion in and of itself, cannot give you strength...

<u>ONLY YOUR RATIONAL THINKING AND PRAYER CAN SAVE YOU FROM SIN!</u>

You can ask for help...but, when you do ask...you must be absolutely sure that you actually want to be helped. Because if you say you are going to change, and you make a promise to either someone else or to yourself to change...you'd better be prepared to suffer the consequences, if you don't.

A word to the wise is sufficient.

MAY GOD BLESS YOUR LOVING SOUL

Chapter 1

Memories

The need for change bulldozed a road
down the center of my mind.

Maya Angelou (1928 - 2014)

[Flashbacks of being a famous singer on stage and then running to a Limousine waiting for me ran through my mind as if it were yesterday...]

The flight attendant's voice seemed to be coming from a thousand miles away as she walked up and down the aisles of the airplane reminding the passengers to buckle their seat belts. The slight tap on my shoulder startled me, and snapped me back to reality.

"I'm sorry to bother you ...Ma'am...We will be landing soon. Please buckle up!" she said to me, speaking in a beautiful English accent.

The breathtaking beauty of the South African landscape drew my attention back to the window for a few more minutes of admiration. I had been planning this trip for months and could hardly believe that one of my fondest dreams was about to come true, finally. The bright sub-equatorial sun glinting off the airplanes and parked cars on the tarmac reminded me of the flashbulbs that used to pop in my face after a big engagement on the road.

Only, those flashes had long since disappeared and were being replaced by the hot flashes of peri-menopause. I truly, was about to embark upon an entirely different phase of my life. I anxiously waited for its unfolding.

My legs felt weak as I tried to stand. The thirteen hour flight had taken its toll on my leg nerves, when I felt the tingling sensations working their way up from my feet to my knees. I plopped back down into my seat and began massaging my calves. The attendant looked concerned.

"I'll be fine...," I explained to her. "...just give me a few seconds."

"I understand, Ma'am...it happens all the time. Take your time."

I don't think she could ever understand the aches and pains of being a middle-aged, "has-been"---she didn't even know who I was. Her perfectly made up, blemish-free face and size four figure struck a chord of slight jealousy in my heart. I was a bit ashamed of myself for feeling that way. Over the years, my own face had gotten much rounder; not to mention my spreading hips and the ever present spare tire around my waist; but I still looked reasonably good for a woman my age.

No one who met me today would have guessed that I was once one of the hottest female singers in the world. Twenty-five years had not only erased any semblance of my former self, but they had also erased the adoration that used to fuel my very existence. My ego took a huge blow when I had to retire.

I walked slowly through the tunnel leading to the terminal, giving my legs more time to recover, thinking about the many times that I had to practically run to my waiting limousine to avoid the screaming throngs of fans and paparazzi. This time it was so very, very different.

The limousine driver that had been sent to pick me up was waiting at the gate with a large placard with my name scrawled on it. It was slightly misspelled; reminding me how difficult my maiden name was to pronounce and that was the reason why I changed it to just my initials in the first place.

I chuckled to myself, as I noticed that he wore a tailored black suit, dark glasses and a crisp white shirt and tie, despite the oppressive heat of the noonday African sun. 'Standard attire, I guess' ; thinking about how good my fiancé, Sly, looked in his black suit when he left for work in the morning.

My driver looked very distinguished as he politely held the door of the car open for me, but he was no Sly. I couldn't help but think about my fiancé and the argument that we had the night before I left.

"Sly, you freaking idiot...I'm going to be gone for two weeks! You should have thought about that *before* you went to the club!"

"Two whole weeks? And, what am I supposed to do with this for two whole weeks while you're away?"

He lifted his t-shirt to show me that he was visibly aroused.

"Stick it up your ass, for all I care. I have a plane to catch in a few hours."

"I can't believe you're gonna just leave me hanging like this!"

"Well, I can't believe you didn't come home until three o'clock in the morning, and *you knew* I was leaving town tomorrow...or today. Oh, you know what I mean! What the hell were you doing all night, anyway...as if I didn't know?"

"My client wanted me to go to another strip bar. What was I supposed to do? Tell him 'no' I don't want to make another $300, Sir. I love being poor!" He tried to explain his financial motivations while climbing into bed next to me.

"Oh, God forbid…you should ever turn down some money---or, the chance to look at another naked stripper's jiggling ass!!"

My soon-to-be-husband had a slight problem with watching pornography and then going to strip clubs on the weekends. We talked about it constantly, but he swore that I was the only woman in the world he wanted to be with, and I believed him. He tried to tell me that the clubs had strict policies about the girls going home with the clients, and that the clients were forbidden to touch the dancers, so I let him have his fun. Besides, he seemed to enjoy having sex with me more when he did come home on time.

He also swore up and down, that he would cut down on going to the clubs as soon as we were married. He promised that he would only take his clients out, and that he would, at least, try to stay in the limo until they were ready to go home. I understood the nature of his job, so as long as he came home on time, and paid our bills like he was supposed to, I couldn't complain, too much.

I am certainly not advocating the porn business, because Lord knows, there are enough problems in the world with child molesters, the rampant spread of AIDS/HIV and the myriad of other sexually transmitted diseases out there.

I would never want anyone in my family, and especially not one of my own daughters, to feel like that was the only way that they could make enough money to survive. Shaking your butt in front of a bunch of horny men and having them throw dollar bills at you on stage, is the same thing as prostitution in my mind.

But, I am not the one to judge---strippers, prostitutes, even their patrons---as long as they stay clean and stay away from *my man*, I am OK with it. They will have to answer to God about their behavior, the same as I will have to answer to Him about mine.

The sight of the handsome limousine driver made me miss my fiancé even more. And, even though he was impeccably dressed, he still carried that distinctive African aroma about him. It was raw and heady.

I thought about pheromones and what makes men and women attractive to one another. Images of sensuously decorated African dancers swarmed in my head, as we pulled under the parking canopy of the hotel where I was to be staying for the next two weeks. I was staring at him intently in the rear view mirror when he finally spoke.

"Here we are, Madame. I hope you enjoy your stay!"

"Oh…I am sure I will!" I answered, while reaching into my handbag to find my wallet for his tip.

"Oh…that won't be necessary," he explained. "The king will be taking care of everything."

"Well now…that's what I'm talking about!" I said, excitedly, as I zipped up my bag and grabbed my belongings off the seat.

I stepped out of the limousine and turned to see a well-dressed woman standing on the curb with a clipboard in her hands. She came towards me with quick steps and bowed slightly. She was dressed in a beautiful white suit made of fine linen. She smiled broadly at me with perfectly straight, white teeth, set in her round, smooth, dark brown face and said:

> "Welcome to Swaziland, Ma'am. My name is Miss Mutala, I am a representative of King Malik, who wishes you a pleasant and exciting stay in our country."

I couldn't believe what I was seeing or hearing. I was being treated like true royalty *on my first trip* to the Motherland. This was a veritable dream come true! My women's entrepreneurial club back in the States had arranged this meeting with the king, who was seeking to develop new joint ventures with burgeoning American businesses to spur the economy in his country. He had picked my interior design business from a thousand other proposals and I was supremely flattered.

At the reception in my honor, on the last day of my stay there, I sat at the king's right elbow as we talked briefly about my life in America.

"What does your husband do for a living?" he asked.

"Oh...I'm not married. Not yet, anyway. My fiancé is a chauffeur," I explained.

"A driver? You are about to marry a common driver?" he chuckled.

"He's *a professional driver*", I said, curtly, and began to feel a little insulted.

"He's a good man and he makes good money. We are doing very well, if I must say so, myself."

"Hmmmph...my wives do not work...and most of the wives of our diplomats here do not work, either."

"Well, I'm sorry, but, most of the women in America have to work, that is, if they want to eat and live indoors!"

His smug attitude was beginning to get on my nerves.

"You would not have to work if you lived, here. A woman of your great beauty, intelligence, and talent would have a life of leisure and comfort. You would be worshiped and have all your needs fulfilled!"

All your needs fulfilled...all your needs fulfilled...the words rang in my ears throughout the entire night while we ate delicious spicy chicken with peanut sauce, steamed rice balls and exotic vegetables. Dessert was French petite fours dipped in rich dark melted chocolate, --- my absolute favorite. We drank pink champagne and listened to a steel band playing what sounded a lot like calypso music.

Before the night was over, a troupe of scantily clad dancers entertained us with their chocolaty gyrations. Their sensuous movements mesmerized me and stirred my passions. At one point during the festivities, the king placed his hand on top of mine, and patted it to the beat of the drums. I was in total Paradise. The champagne was making my head swim and, sadly enough, jet lag was also beginning to set in.

No one even batted an eye when the king nodded to his personal guards, grabbed me by the hand, and led me to the lobby of the reception hall with his guards following closely behind us.

"Miss C.J., you look very tired, please--- let me escort you back to your room, personally."

He led me by my elbow to the bank of elevators and pushed the button on the wall. I hardly realized what was happening until we were inside the hotel suite's vestibule. I was definitely drunk and a little bit out of my mind.

"Hey, wait a minute…this isn't my room," I said, with my speech slurring slightly.

"No,---my naïve visitor. This is a glimpse into your future. The best is yet to come."

I looked around and almost fainted from the sight of the opulent decorations of the king's suite. He kissed my hand gently, and pulled me towards the huge bed with the gold satin spread. I started to shake my head in protest.

"No...I can't do this..." I begged him, and tried to pull away.

He put his finger gently over my lips.

"Yes, you can...with this," he said softly, grabbed one of my hands and placed it on his private parts. "Your fiancé could never take care of you, like I could, my precious one. That is why I brought you here, Miss C.J.,--- I want you to be with me forever."

He bent down slightly and slowly kissed my forehead. He moved to my lips and his kisses were sweet and gentle. My head was spinning more now as his hands roamed all over my body. My thoughts were racing...

'What about Sly? What about Sly!! He doesn't own a country, girl...He hasn't even paid for his own car! Why do you stay with that Buster, anyway?... Why do you stay with that Buster, anyway? ... You're going to marry a common

**driver...a common driver...a common driver?... All
your needs would be fulfilled...fulfilled....fulfilled!"**

The next few moments seemed to pass in slow
motion. Our clothing came off quickly and King Malik
kissed me all over my body...my neck, my breasts, my
abdomen... places my fiancé never attempted to explore.
His natural odors were exciting me even more. I wanted
him inside of me. My good senses flew out the window
and all I could feel was dampness, sweat, and my private
parts pulsating wildly.

"Wait a minute," I said, suddenly. "We can't do
this, like this...I mean,...don't we need to use a
condom?"

"Oh no, my sweet queen-to-be...we do not use
condoms here. They destroy the true feelings,"
the king explained, and kept thrusting inside of
me.

"No, no...please," I begged. "You have to stop, or
else you're gonna *have to* put on a condom."

14

Reluctantly and slowly, he got up and went to the door. A few moments later he returned to the side of the bed with a small golden foil packet in his hand. He opened it with his teeth and began the arduous task of putting on the contents.

"Your guards keep your condoms?"

"Just in case...What would it look like, ...a king carrying condoms around in his wallet?"

The rest of the night was a virtual blur, and the most intense experience of my life. I started to feel a little guilty about Sly, but it was way too late for me to stop. I kept thinking about what the king had said to me earlier in the evening, and it made me even more excited. He wanted me to be with him forever!

He was an expert lover and, after he had climaxed, he immediately got up and went into the bathroom. He returned with a warm washcloth to clean my pubic area for me. Then, without saying another word, he dressed quickly, kissed me on my forehead again,and left the room.

I was so exhausted that I turned over in that huge bed and fell asleep, sucking my thumb like a little baby. I think I had a dream about riding in a big pink Cadillac convertible, wearing a flowing white gauze dress, and waving to a crowd of adoring followers.

The next morning I stumbled to the bathroom and as I was sitting on the toilet, I noticed something in the trash basket. There at the bottom of the basket was the condom that the king had used, obviously torn to bits. I suddenly, felt very nauseous.

I barely had time to think about what I should do next. I had to catch my plane back home in a couple of hours and couldn't start making phone calls to the palace. Besides, I was a willing participant in the activities, what could I possibly say to the authorities? I didn't even have a phone number to call him, directly.

I kept thinking about how stupid I was for allowing myself to get so drunk that I wasn't in control of my faculties for rational thinking. I simply decided to keep it a secret. I would never tell anyone what had happened to me that night, and I would file the incident away in my **"Oh Damn --- I Messed Up Again!"** portfolio. I pulled out my day planner PDA and made a quick note to myself to be sure to make an appointment at the doctor when I got back to the States for an HIV blood test. What else could I do?

The damage had already been done.

Chapter 2

Misery

A wretched soul, bruised with adversity, We bid be
quiet when we hear it cry; But were we burdened with
like weight of pain, as much or more we should
ourselves complain.

William Shakespeare (1564-1616)

I hated the thought of having to drive back to
New York in a rented car, almost as much as I hated the
thought of seeing my dysfunctional relatives pretending
to be a loving family at one of the worst times of my life,
again. They always managed to peel back the layers of
plastic covering their hearts anytime someone in the
family passed away, but at any other time, they were as
hard and cold as the one thousand miles of pavement
that lay ahead of me. Like my little cousin used to say:

"We'll see you the next time somebody dies!"

I tried to not think about the pains that shot through my solar-plexus every time I thought about spending more than a few perfunctory minutes around the bunch of misfits and ne'er-do-wells that we called "our people," and I began to focus on the Stevie Wonder song that was playing on the radio.

"As around the sun the earth knows she's revolving..."

Where the Hell were they while I was lying in that flea bag motel with the sounds of prostitutes taking care of business in the next room keeping me up at night, and the drug dealers bothering me with all their cat calls; constantly giving me the heads-up to come buy their products whenever I walked from my car in the evening, especially if they thought I had money, just because I was driving a Mercedes?

The tears started to well up in my eyes as I tried to maintain control of the car and focus on the white lines shooting past the hood in front of me. I sang along with Stevie, and for a few fleeting moments I pretended to be back on stage, doing all the background parts in perfect harmony. I started to forget all about my stomach pains.

But then, my heart skipped three beats the second the sound of the siren and the flashing lights coming from the parked State Trooper's car on the side of the road shook me from my pain-induced stupor.

'Got-dammit!!' I thought. 'Why did he have to pick me out of all the other cars traveling right along with me?'

My niece, Darette, awoke from her morning nap when she felt me brake suddenly, as I pulled to the shoulder of the highway. She proclaimed sleepily:

"I told you, you can't go speeding through 'Sous Cakalaki', Auntie! They will catch you every time!"

I needed another speeding ticket like I needed a bullet hole in my already finance-riddled pocketbook.

"License and registration, please…" said the stern-faced officer, as he quickly surveyed the contents and passengers of my van.

My son, Milo complained briefly that we had interrupted his video game. But, he soon calmed down when he realized that we had been stopped by a police officer, and that I wasn't just pulling over for another quick pit stop, again.

"Please, officer…" I begged; trying to get a minutia of sympathy out of a man who had already heard every excuse in the book. "…I am on my way to my mother's funeral in New York and I am already late."

Only this time…*I was telling the truth!*

"Yeah, well…now that explains why you were going thirty miles an hour over the speed limit, now don't it?" he said, sarcastically, as he walked around to the back of the car to get the license plate number and then back to my open window.

After he took my driver's license and registration numbers, he gingerly handed me the yellow ticket ripped from his clipboard.

"Have a nice trip, and slow down, Lady!" he said with a big smile on his face as he walked back to his squad car.

"Damn...he didn't even act like he cared, did he, Auntie?" Darette said, angrily.

"You got that right--- the damned pig!" I added, as I shook my head in disbelief, threw the ticket into the console, and slowly pulled the van back onto the highway.

"How are you gonna explain that one to Sly?" she said curiously.

"I don't have to explain nothing to nobody. Sly don't run my life. And, besides...he has to take a trip to California this week and he's gonna be gone for three whole months, so I got some time to get the money together or else fight it out of court."

I explained this to her knowing full well that my darling husband was going to find out, sooner or later, that I had destroyed our monthly budget once again, and he would probably give me some major grief about it later on. I knew that I had some bad spending habits. But, in my mind I was still single, and it was mostly my money. I had to get used to being married again.

"Why do you stay with that fool anyway? And, why didn't he come with us to attend Grandma's funeral? I'd leave his ignorant ass as soon as we get back to Atlanta if I were you---the cold-hearted mother-f___er."

"Maybe I will," I answered her, curtly. "The bastard didn't even stick around long enough this morning to say goodbye to me. He just got ready for work as usual and left at 5:30 A.M.. He thinks the world revolves around that stupid limousine business. I'm so sorry I convinced him to go independent and get away from that old company he was working for.

He's making a boatload of money, but he's spending less and less time with me. It's just plain disgusting."

Sylvester Greene had asked me to be his wife just a few short months before I found out that my mother was dying of Cancer. I hesitated to go through with the ceremony without my mother's blessing, but since she had slipped into a drug-induced coma and remained there for four months after the doctors found the tumors on her uterus, and started an extremely aggressive form of chemotherapy on her already weakened body, there was no way that she could have been there for me. We knew in our hearts that it was just a matter of time before the inevitable was going to happen.

The knowledge that my mother was going to die put an inordinate strain on our relationship and I had wanted to cancel everything because, after all, we had only been dating for a few months when I had brought up the subject of marriage. But, it was Sly who insisted that we go through with the ceremony, claiming that I would never return to Atlanta if I went back to New York to be with my mother. He didn't want to leave Atlanta and he wanted to keep me as close to him as possible, especially since he knew that I was closer to my family than he was to his.

It felt weird not having Mommy or anyone from my family by my side as I said my wedding vows in front of the judge downtown at the Atlanta City Hall. I had dreams of a big church ceremony with the expensive designer gown my whole life, and had to settle for a civil ceremony with another white evening suit from Rich's, when I realized that at 45 years old, it was probably going to be my last chance to find a man to marry me.

"You know the man shortage ain't gonna get no better..." My best friend, Cynthia Taylor, reminded me when I hesitated to sign the marriage registration papers just two weeks before the ceremony.

"Shoot…Sly ain't no Denzel…but, he sho' ain't no Quasimodo, either. You'd better marry that man before his old girlfriend gets wind that he's finally asked you and she tries to get him back!"

Well, it all began when I planned a night out on the town with my colleagues and ordered a limousine to impress one of the new girls with the company.

> "Man, Miss C.J. you sure do know how to treat your employees, right!" said the new girl, Verona Thompkins, as she stepped into the long, white stretch limo.
>
> "O-o-o-weeee! This thing is sweeeeet!!
>
> "Dang…It's got colored lights and everything!" Cynthia chimed in.
>
> "Girls…you are working for the best little company in Atlanta. But, there is nothing little about the way that I do business," I boasted. "You see I got the best limo company and one of their best drivers tonight. Isn't that right, Sly?"

26

Sly had merely nodded and smiled his most beautiful professional smile; not wanting to fraternize too much with his clients, because he knew it was against the company's rules to do so. But, I caught him looking in the rear view mirror several times that night and shared a knowing nod of the head between us.

After we dropped all the other girls off, he and I talked for a few minutes outside of my house. The smell of his cologne was intoxicating as I tried to concentrate on the conversation and not the size of the bulge that was visibly growing in his trousers. I gave him my business card and the rest is history. He waited a few days to make that first call, but soon he was calling me practically every day.

I guess you could say that both he and I were on the rebound when we first met. I certainly wasn't looking for love and couldn't have cared less if I had ever found another man. I was focusing on my business career --- not romance. Sly had just broken up with his girlfriend of three years over two thousand dollars that she had stolen from his bank account, and he didn't want to get involved with another woman so quickly.

Therefore, I assured him that I didn't want, nor did I need his money, as the settlement from my divorce kept me in the designer boutiques, often enough. The fact that I was an independently wealthy divorcée appealed to him immensely, especially since he had plans to go into business for himself, and didn't need another gold-digging albatross hanging around his neck.

It took a while for us to actually go on a date. At first we just talked on the phone, because he didn't have much free time and neither did I. I truly wanted a real friend, and not just another quick roll in the sack as we "old heads" used to say.

Sly wasn't much to look at, but he had a winning personality and I just loved his smooth, chocolaty brown skin and "teddy bear" figure. I was tired of all the pretty boy, upwardly mobile, workout obsessed, executive types who had floated in and out of my life and needed someone who was a little more down to earth. He didn't live in a big house, and didn't drive the latest model Benz or even a big SUV.

He lived in a condo that he had owned for over seven years, worked for a prestigious limo company for over ten years, and drove a Volvo. He wasn't on drugs, hadn't been incarcerated (at least not in the last 10 years) and didn't beat his women. He was 100% percent better in bed than my last boyfriend and he didn't ask me for money all the time.

The first time we made love I felt an instant connection and knew that he was going to be in my life for a very long time. His only faults were that he smoked weed and he liked to watch porno videos. But, most single men watch porno so they don't forget what a woman looks like down there, especially if they haven't dated in a long time.

And, I used to smoke weed myself, because I thought that it made me more creative for my artwork, so, as long as Sly didn't do it around me or in the house, I was cool with it. He represented stability, if nothing else, in my mind. He worked hard at what he did and he made a good living.

He wanted to be an independent businessman and knew the value of being a legitimate entrepreneur like myself. He didn't ask me for the money to start his business, he just told me his dreams and I made them happen for him. As far as I knew, he loved me with all of his heart.

At least that is what he told me all of the time while we were dating. We were good together. Or, so I believed. One thing I could say about me and Sly, we trusted one another. Because without trust we knew that we had nothing. So, when we signed those papers we knew that we were putting our lives into each other's hands...forever.

That didn't mean that we never lied to one another, it just meant that we kept our secrets to ourselves in the hopes that no one would find out and no one would get hurt in the long run. But, things began to deteriorate between us quickly, when we realized that my mother was actually going to die. Sly couldn't handle my emotional outbreaks after we found out that her illness had worsened and he retreated into his own little world. He just wasn't used to "feeling" things so deeply.

He did things from habit, like working twelve hours a day and sleeping the other ten, eating his dinner at seven o'clock on the nose, playing video games until 1 A.M. and then falling asleep in my arms after we had made love. The ink was barely dry on the marriage certificate, so there was no way we were going to get a divorce.

His days off were dedicated to catching up on his sleep, and my days off were used for getting caught up with the housework or putting a dent in the backlog of paperwork that had piled up after my last trip to New York, Los Angeles, Chicago or Africa. We were the proverbial ships passing in the night; though longing to connect again, but not knowing how or when. We were independent souls trying to make a go of a marriage that maybe should never have happened.

I had to pay for my daughter's humongous college tuition that month, along with my son's private school fees, put a large payment on my mother's nursing home care bill, and to make matters worse, my car had recently been repossessed for a couple of late payments. I had run through my settlement like sand through a sieve, setting up Sly in his limousine business, flying back and forth across the country, traveling to Africa, paying for nannies and babysitters to take care of my ten year old son Milo, and buying one too many pairs of Louis Vuitton shoes.

Our money was tight and Sly's fists were even tighter when it came to giving me anything other than my weekly spending allowance. This trip to attend my mother's funeral would prove to be the infamous straw that broke the camel's back. We could never have dreamed what was going to happen to us.

"You know that Sly is gonna wring your pretty little neck when he finds out about that one hundred and sixty-five dollar speeding ticket.

You know that he don't care about nothing except how much money you're spending on this trip."

My niece's observations cut me to the quick.

"My husband loves me!" was my quick retort, as Darette looked at me sideways in disbelief.

"Yeah, but do you love him?"

That was the question that I could not answer.

Sylvester Greene was a very strange character. He didn't allow people inside his head, his bed, his house, or his heart too often. His rough exterior and abrasive nature hid a heart of gold and a vulnerability that he tried to pretend did not exist. He had a terrible secret that even I could not wrangle out of him; a secret that made him grind his teeth, jump up out of his sleep, and scream out in terror in the wee hours of the morning.

Every time it happened and I asked him about it, he would tell me that is was just a nightmare about Viet Nam. He had served two years on the Mekong Delta, and the memories of his time overseas haunted him miserably. But, something told me it was much deeper than mere shell shock. He adamantly refused to see a doctor and my suggestions to talk to one were met with stern indignation. He was definitely, as stubborn and set in his ways, as an old farmyard goat.

He had vowed undying love to me, though, especially since I was the one who had paid for our wedding, our home in the suburbs, his business and practically everything else that we shared. He was a good businessman, as far as I knew, but he had a short fuse when it came to the way that I spent money. I was good at knowing what to spend it on, but, not too savvy about saving or investing it. He knew that keeping tabs on our credit cards and paying bills on time, was not my strong suit.

We had agreed that although the major portion of the bank accounts was technically *my money*. When we got married it became *our money*. And he, being *the man*, I gave him the respect that he would be the one in control of the family assets.

So, when the bank called to demand payment on my Mercedes, he wasn't shocked, but he was very angry that I had not paid the bill on time.

"I told you to take care of that, now didn't I? Didn't I?" He had said sternly; reprimanding me like he was a dutiful parent.

"I was waiting for one of my customers to pay me... and I couldn't get the money to the bank on time," I had said, trying to defend my negligent actions.

"You couldn't have asked them for an extension, C.J.?"

"That was the extension..."

"You mean to tell me you've missed more than one payment?"

"It's been a bad month for my business...what can I tell you?"

"You can tell me that you paid my limo bill on time." He said, dryly.

"Of course, I did, Honey…"

I had lied; hoping that the check that I had just written to the limo financing company wouldn't bounce before I got back from New York. I had planned to ask my big brother, Antoine, to cover me for the payments until my client paid me, because we had just enough money in the bank to cover our mortgage, some of the monthly utility bills and the rental car fees on the credit card.

Our bills added up to just a little over five thousand dollars a month, and although his limousine business was doing well, and my design business was developing, we still needed to keep tabs on our money. We managed to keep up a good front for the neighbors, but the truth of the matter was that we were technically broke. Filing for bankruptcy was not an option, and we struggled monthly to keep up the façade of wealth and privilege.

My money was tied up in what few investments I had made when my settlement finally did come through, but basically we were cash poor like so many other millionaires out there. I was not used to living on a budget, and Sly was the one who guarded the checkbooks like a C.O. guarding prison gates.

I needed to find a way to get my life back on track. I loved my husband but the stress of dealing with our money problems was beginning to take its toll on our marriage. Money problems can destroy a relationship quicker than infidelity, illness or a crime. Very few marriages can survive a change in the financial status of the partners, and we were about to be tested beyond the limits of human endurance in relation to how important money, health, and trust (or the lack, thereof) was to the two of us and a few other people in our lives. The lies that we had told to one another and the ones we were going to tell were about to catch up to us in a very bad way.

Chapter 3

Pleasantry

A handful of patience is worth more

than a bushel of brains.

A Dutch Proverb

"Wake up, Darette...we're almost to Virginia and it's your turn to drive!"

I didn't have the heart to wake my niece up sooner. Besides, when I took those long trips home, I liked to get the road behind me, so to speak. Darette wasn't exactly the best driver in the world either, and I feared for our lives coming through the mountains in North Carolina. So, I let her sleep most of the trip; expecting to catch a few hours of sleep for myself before we got to New York. We pulled into a gas station in Roanoke, Virginia to fill up for the last leg of the trip. Darette got behind the wheel and immediately lit up a cigarette.

"Keep the window cracked...," I reminded her. "...you know I can't stand those nasty things."

"Oh, Auntie...*you know* that I have a nervous condition and I have to light up *something*. I can't fire up a joint with you-know-who in the backseat."

"Those things stink, anyway..." my son complained and covered up his nose with his shirt. "...and, the smoke hurts my eyes."

"Well...they don't hurt *my eyes* and you need to just shut up," she said.

"Look, you just keep *your eyes* on the road, Missy, get us there in one piece, and stop talking to my kid like that," I scolded her in my most motherly tone.

Not having any of her own, and having no intentions of ever having any, Darette had absolutely no patience with children. Although she was almost forty

39

years old, she acted more like a regressed teenager herself. She did whatever she could get away with.

"Remember... we need to stop in Jersey to fill up again so we won't be coming through the city on empty, and have to pay those crazy New York prices for gas," I reminded her before I got ready to konk out.

She assured me that she wouldn't forget and agreed to pay her share of the gas bill so I wouldn't have to dip back into my pocketbook again unnecessarily. I adjusted my seat into the reclining position, put my pillow behind my head and stretched out my legs to rest my aching body from the long nine hours that I had just driven. Five hours later, I felt the car jerk to a stop and I awoke with the bright lights of a gas station blaring in my face. We were just outside of New York City at a rest stop on the Pennsylvania Turnpike.

"Auntie, wake up it's your turn to drive!"

"What do you mean...my turn?" I looked at my watch and it said 11 pm. "You've only been driving and I've only been sleeping for five hours. I'm exhausted!"

"But, Auntie...I don't know my way through New York City."

"What are you talking about? You are thirty-seven years old, you've lived in New York most of your life, you've been back and forth to Georgia a bunch of times. What do you mean, you don't know your way through the city?"

"We always came through Staten Island...I don't know this way," she said with a face as serious as a heart attack.

Oh my God! I felt like wringing her neck. If I wasn't so patient and so broke, I would have left her at the gas station with money to take the bus home. Instead, I walked inside the snack shop to get a cup of coffee and buy a Lotto ticket. The flashing lights of the Lotto machine read: **"300 Million Dollars"**

'Boy what I could do with some money like that, right now,' I thought, as the attendant wished me luck and handed me the small pink and white ticket along with my change. I threw the ticket into my purse and walked back to my car. I was still pissed at Darette.

"Bitch...you are lucky you are family..." I said to Darette, as I climbed behind the wheel of the van. "...'cause I am about to commit murder right about now!"

"Aw...come on, Auntie...don't be mad. I'm sooorry..." Darette always used that whiny little voice to get someone's sympathy when she knew she was wrong. The voice got to me every time.

Two hours later, we were stuck in traffic on the George Washington Bridge and still had another hour to go to get to my mother's house on Long Island. My shoulders hurt, my back was tight, my nerves were on edge from the caffeine in the coffee I had just drank, and all I could think about was how I could dispose of my niece's body without getting caught.

Some fool had broken down on the Cross Bronx Expressway in their raggedy old car and had the whole West side of New York in knots. Besides that, they were doing road construction and some a---hole had run over one of those orange cones that they put around the work sites and the thing had exploded under his car. The traffic was backed up to New Jersey.

By the time we had reached my mother's house it was almost three A.M., and luckily my daughter had left the door open for us. I was so exhausted that I couldn't even get out of the car. My niece and my son went inside. I grabbed a blanket and a pillow and fell back asleep in the car.

The next morning, my oldest daughter Marcella, knocked on the window of the car to wake me up.

"Hey....Old Lady! Open the door and give me my hug!"

I rolled down the window and pulled her head to mine. I planted one of those big fat raspberry farts on the side of her face and spit went flying all over the place. I forgot that I hadn't brushed my teeth in over 24 hours.

"Damn, woman…did ya have to let the dragon loose so *early* in the morning? You need a breath mint, bad! "

God, …I truly loved my family to death…the little part that was just mine, that is. The sun rose and set in my children's eyes. My moving to Atlanta had been hard on all of us, but I had to get away or else I would have lost my mind. The years of fighting my ex-husband in court had taken its toll, and at the time, I needed get my life in gear. It had been only two years since my divorce had been finalized and I was struggling to maintain my own place in New York. My ex was getting negligent with the alimony payments and the lawyers were still working out the details of my full settlement.

My singing career had virtually ended many years ago, and Atlanta presented the opportunity for me to find happiness and stability, once and for all. But, I always missed my babies terribly, every time I went away.

"You look good, Mommy…Come on inside and say 'Hi' to your granddaughter--- she's been waiting for you."

It always felt so good to come home. My mother's house was the only place on earth that I could always be myself. I didn't have to pretend to be anybody special, and I didn't have to always be on my guard. The paparazzi hadn't found out about my mother's death, and they hadn't caught up to me yet, otherwise, I wouldn't have come. My home town was off limits to the media hounds, and I made absolutely sure that my assistant knew to come up with a creative excuse for why I had to leave Atlanta so suddenly.

This was definitely not one of those times that I wanted to have my picture taken. I pulled myself out of my blankets, walked towards the house and my granddaughter met me at the door. My butt hurt from sitting down so long.

Nammy…Nammy! You're here!"

Darice was just about nine years old, but she was built solid as a brick house and looked more like she was ten or twelve. She and Milo were just a few months apart in age and were raised to be more like brother and sister. I know it was hard on her when we moved to Atlanta but we kept in touch regularly over the phone and through video conferencing on the computer. She ran to me and nearly knocked me over with her exuberance.

"Hey, Sunshine!" I greeted her with a big hug, and we began to sing together.

"You are my sunshine, my only sunshine. You make me happy when skies are gray..."

"How's your school work, baby?"

"Oh, Nammy...Now don't start with the investigations, already. Come on and have some breakfast with me. I can't wait for you to tell me about your trip to Africa!"

46

"Well now, *that story* is going to have to wait, Darlin'. Because right now, I have to go take a shower, brush my teeth, change my funky clothing and then I will tell you all about it."

My daughter came into the room behind me with a sly smirk on her face.

"Guess who came by here yesterday to give you his condolences, Mommy?"

"Who? The King of Swaziland wants me to come back to be the Queen, already?"

"Don't try to be so funny…You don't have the talent," she began. "Your old boyfriend, Duke Preston, he came here last night and said he was coming to the funeral tomorrow."

"Duke Preston…? Oh my God! I haven't heard that name in twenty-five years."

Duke was my first love. You know--- the first boy to *actually say* that he loved me, sincerely. All the other boys just wanted to get with me because I was a cheerleader. There was this rumor going around that I was supposed to have had sex with every guy on the football team, except that little scrawny water boy mascot. The truth was that I had just dated the quarterback, but nothing serious had ever happened between us.

Nice girls didn't give up the booty so easily back in those days, and I had to protect my reputation as being a decent girl. But, you know boys...they will exaggerate to make themselves look like a Super Stud. And, a guy who is built like Mr. America dating a girl who could do a split jump and touch the back of her head with both of her feet, could conjure up a whole host of juicy gossip. It was just gossip, though. Duke didn't care about the rumors, he just needed someone to love and to cherish him, badly.

"He left his number...you gonna call him back?" she asked.

"Of course, I'm going to call him back! I'm not going to be rude. Duke and I are cool now. It's been a long time. I think I've forgiven him by now."

"But, Mommy...*you know* what'll happen if you see Duke again..." she started to warn me. "Have you forgotten what he did to you?"

"What? You think that I am going to get all warm and fuzzy inside and desecrate my marriage vows? Or, maybe he will go off on the preacher and start something. Please! We are too old for that kind of stuff, girl."

The truth was that Duke had vowed to get me back even if he had to die trying. That kind of love is scary. That was the reason why we had to break up in the first place. He was way too controlling and extremely jealous. He wouldn't even let me *look* at another boy and he would threaten to kill himself every time I even acted like I was going to leave him. Finally, after three years of that nonsense I had to tell him that I couldn't take it anymore and that the relationship was totally over.

Luckily, I was about to go off to college in Connecticut and would've been too far away for him to try to actually get me back. He didn't have the nerve or the gumption to come all the way to another state, but, we had to serve him with papers when he started stalking my mother, and begging her to persuade me to take him back. Eventually he calmed down, found another girlfriend, got married himself, and even had a couple of little Dukes over the years. But, he hung on for a long time after our initial breakup and made a virtual nuisance of himself.

The thought of seeing him again did precipitate a feeling of dread, and uneasiness in my heart. After all, he was the man who had introduced me to The Art of the Kama Sutra; and passing that information on to my boyfriends was a prerequisite for any relationship that I wanted to develop in my life. It was what made my first husband propose to me, because he said that he had never experienced anything like it in his entire life, and didn't want to lose the woman who had taught the techniques to him.

Duke and I were just eighteen years old when he had started studying Eastern philosophy and yoga. It was in the summer, right after our high school graduation, that he had found this book on the art of lovemaking to raise your spiritual consciousness, and decided that we were "grown" enough to experiment with the principals taught in the book. One night after we had spent hours changing positions, suppressing climax after climax, and then finally collapsing exhausted from one gigantic orgasm, Duke swore that I was going to be his woman forever. We were together nearly every day after that.

But then, it was hard for Duke to let go when our relationship began to deteriorate, because he had lost his own mother to cancer at such a very young age and didn't have the love of a good female in his life. His father was an alcoholic, and his step-mother was the neighborhood prostitute. He had idolized his mother, who was a Sunday school teacher and a nurse; the exact opposite of his father's second wife, who basically ignored him and spent most of her time shopping for new clothing, and potential customers.

He clung to anyone and anything that represented love and affection to him. I just couldn't give him what he needed because I had my own demons to deal with. I had secrets that I had never told anyone in my life.

My own parents had divorced when I was a very young child and I don't remember much about my real father. He died when I was about eight years old and my mother had remarried shortly thereafter, but she didn't tell me who he was, or that he was dead until I was almost seventeen and the fact that she had kept the secret from me for such a long time put a wedge between us over the years. My step-father was a very cold and distant alcoholic who turned out to be a closet homosexual, and I longed for the loving attention of a man in my life.

It was this common thread in our lives that bonded me to Duke. He had filled the void in me for a while, until my senior year of high school when I lost thirty pounds, went out for the cheering squad and became one of the most popular girls in the school. After dating the guy on the football team, I ended up with Duke and for three years we were inseparable. Deep down inside I truly did love him.

My daughter caught me by the arm as I headed for the bathroom.

"Where is Sly...I thought he was coming with you?" she asked.

"No...um...there's a couple of big awards shows coming up in Los Angeles and he's going to help out a buddy of his get set up in the limousine business. He sends his condolences, though."

"His condolences?" her voice got high and shrill. "His condolences? You mean to tell me he couldn't postpone his trip for *one day* to be with his wife at the worst time of her life? What kind of Buster did you marry, anyway?"

"It's three days…and Sly is not a Buster…he's a very loving and supportive man," I countered.

"Save the bull for your fans, Miss C.J.…*this is me, Marcy,* that you're talking to. Remember…the one you call on the phone to talk about all the times he's left you lonely and embarrassed?"

"I don't know what you're talking about…"

"Go on and take your shower…maybe the hot water will help you get your memory back, --- Queen of De-nial! Maybe *you should* go on back to Africa and be with the King. I think you left your brains there, anyway," she taunted me sarcastically.

Unfortunately, she was right. Sly and I hadn't been getting along lately. We hardly talked anymore and we were either too busy or too tired to have sex. I think it had been over six weeks since the last time we had physical relations, and I really needed to feel loved again. Deep down inside, I was truly afraid to see Duke again and I never did call him back. I got busy with the preparations for my mother's funeral and tried to forget about seeing him.

Chapter 4

Respectfully

Although the world is full of suffering, it is full also of the overcoming of it.

Helen Keller (1880 - 1968)

Why is it that every time you get around your relatives you become a totally different person? Or, maybe *the real you* has a tendency to come out? Anyway, with me...I always turned into this shy, totally reticent, wallflower type who has absolutely nothing in common with "my people" except to share some genetic material. And, my relatives have a tendency to always put on that plastered-smile game face that *you know* is hiding a load of crap bigger than Mount Everest. The only person in my family who was truly, truly "real" was my Aunt Jillian.

"Girl you look fatter and fatter every time I see you…"

"Auntie…I'm forty-six years old now…I'm supposed to look fat."

"Yeah, but you ain't *never* gonna find a man looking like that."

"Auntie…*I am married now*. Remember,--- I married Sylvester Greene in February?"

"Sly-vester who? Oh yeah, --- the taxi driver."

"No, Auntie…he's a professional chauffeur."

"Taxi driver…chauff-ooor…jitney driver… whatever *you* want to call him…He still picks up people in a car and drives them around, right?. When are you gonna find someone who's got *a real job* in an office or something? Where is he anyway? He should be here with you! What kind of husband leaves his wife to attend her mother's funeral alone?"

It was no use trying to explain anything to her. She was 82 years old, half deaf, half blind, and mean as a hornet. She'd forget her own name if we didn't have to call her fifty times to get her attention. She'd put five husbands in the ground in her life and lately she couldn't give a rats behind who got married, divorced, or murdered in our family. All she cared about was whether or not my cousin was going to take her to play Bingo on Friday nights at the local firehouse.

She used to be an extremely beautiful woman, with a hot, tight body and long flowing curls that swept her perfectly made up face like a model's. She could put Lena Horne to shame back in the day and was still very good looking for her age. Men would practically fall at her feet and she had her pick of all the local eligible bachelors, but she was truly a one man woman. If only her one man could stay alive long enough to keep her happy. It seemed like every time she'd married a new one, he would drop dead from some unexplained illness a few years later.

We never did find out why they kept dropping like flies. They never found anything suspicious in my dead uncles' bodies, and she never went to jail, so I guess she had the "ill na-na", for real! We used to tease her about it, but now she is content to call herself the "Real Black Widow," and that doesn't stop the guys at the bingo hall from flocking around her when she comes to play, either.

She walks in that place with her thirty year old mink coat, her support stockings rolled up under her Gloria Vanderbilt skirt suit with the satin collar, smelling like Chanel #5 and the old guys melt like butter on a hot griddle. She had her pick of suitors, even at the ripe old age of eighty-two.

My mother was practically the exact opposite of her sister. Where my auntie was the vivacious social butterfly, my mother was more the shy and retiring homebody. Her family was her life, and she dedicated herself to providing a nice home and a good life for her children. Her only downfall was the fact that she had married the wrong man; a man who had vowed, not to love and respect her forever, but to ruin her for life.

He was jealous of her many accomplishments and became a shameful alcoholic over the years. He embarrassed her at every opportunity and every political function became a tedious disaster. He eventually became very ill, struggled with cirrhosis of the liver, and died of emphysema at the age of seventy.

She didn't cry at his funeral. On the contrary, she called it a "sweet relief" that he was no longer suffering and neither was she. She went on to become a successful businesswoman and community advocate until too much stress, and too many family problems had contributed to the cancer that eventually took her life a month short of her eightieth birthday.

She had come to hate what the world had become with its political corruption and moral decline, and she longed for the simpler times of her youth. Her body had become weakened from age and the pain of the cancer. I thought that her death was the "sweet relief" that she had needed in the twilight years of her life.

I was like my mother in a lot of ways. I looked a lot like her and we shared a lot of the same views on Life. She would beg me to not make the same bad choices that she had made in her life and I vowed to not do so. However, sometimes we are destined to repeat history, so to speak, unless we actually take heed and learn the lessons of our forefathers, (or mothers as the case may be).

I didn't cry when I found out that she had died. Again, all I could think about was the 'sweet relief' and the fact that she was no longer suffering. I held in my feelings and presented a façade of strength and poise. But, deep down inside...I was dying, too.

Mother had been cremated and we had decided to give her a memorial ceremony instead of a traditional funeral so the tone and mood of the service was a little bit lighter and less depressing than usual. My Uncle Theodore was a consummate preacher, with a wry sense of humor, who had everyone in stitches as he gave the eulogy for my mother. It made the time go faster and cheered us up, so we thought that we were at the local comedy club instead of a funeral. At the end of his service, he invited members of the family and the community to come up to the podium and share their memories of my mother.

Of course we had our share of drug addicts, prostitutes, criminals and adulterers in the family, but the only difference was...we pretended that they didn't exist. Anyone who had a checkered past just became the topic of hushed tones, and whispered conversations shared between family members or friends who knew what the deal was in the family. We always kept up the air of respectability at all cost.

So, after about an hour into the ceremony when my niece and two cousins came staggering into the building, wreaking of alcohol and weed, pushing past all the people who had been standing in the hallways and the aisles of the funeral home to take their places in the section reserved for our immediate family, everyone's tongues started wagging like crazy.

"Some of us have their own agendas," began my cousin Josephine, who was standing at the podium giving her comments:

"Some of us need to be reminded that life is short and that you never know when it's going to be your turn next."

"And, some of us need to mind their own damned business..." Darette remarked, just loud enough for those of us sitting in the front row of seats to hear her.

Now, Josephine weighed about three hundred pounds and did not take any guff from anyone. Her demeanor changed immediately and her fists tightened visibly. She and Darette were not on the best of terms, because Darette used to buy weed from Josephine's husband, hung around their house until all hours of the morning, and one night Josephine had caught them getting ready to get busy on her living room couch and kicked Darette out of her house in her underwear.

Josephine had started to come from behind the podium when Uncle Teddy grabbed her by the shoulders.

"And, some of us need to learn that there is a time and a place for everything…and, *now is not the time nor the place* to air our differences," he reminded Josephine, who bit her bottom lip and took a deep breath. "It is the time to remember my dear sister and how she would have wanted us to handle our differences."

"My aunt was a saint,…" Josephine began again. "…unlike some *other people* we know, she led an exemplary life."

"What the hell is exemplary? Speak English woman!" Darette yelled from her seat in the corner.

Darette couldn't resist being the center of attention especially when she was drunk, which she obviously was drunk *and high as a kite* at that moment.

"That's it...I can't take it anymore!!" Josephine yelled, as she let go of the microphone and rounded the podium as quickly as her three hundred pounds would let her move.

She had almost made it to the section where Darette, who was now standing with her hands raised in the air ready to fight (or to get her butt kicked!), when Uncle Teddy caught up to her.

"Let go of the fat bitch...she can't hurt me!" Darette taunted. *"Let her go!"*

The other grandchildren were trying to get her to sit down without success.

This time he didn't quite get a hold of her as tightly as he should have, and Josephine shook him off like a quarterback shaking off a lineman going for the long pass. Uncle Teddy's hip hit the table where my mother ashes sat in a tall silver urn, and the urn went flying across the table; spreading my mother's ashes all over the carpeting like so much fertilizer on a grassy lawn.

The whole congregation gasped simultaneously.
Auntie Jillian fainted. My oldest sister, Sanai, who was
sitting in the front row, jumped up quickly and managed
to cut off my cousin before she could reach the other side
of the pulpit. Josephine stopped dead in her tracks at the
sight of another big woman standing right in front of her
waving her arms like a defending point guard. Sanai put
her arms down and spoke angrily:

> **"Could we please...stop showing our behinds
> and, start showing some class for a change?**
> For once in your life, could you just forget the past,
> woman? Your husband left you because you
> gained two hundred pounds! I would have cheated
> on your fat behind, too! For God's sake, girl, let it
> go!!!"

Practically everyone covered their mouths and
snickered. A distinct murmur of laughter went through
the crowd and my uncle called for order and quiet.
Josephine turned to go back to the podium to continue
her speech as my uncle composed his self, and apologized
profusely for knocking over Momma's urn. He called for

a Dust buster, and soon the ceremony was back on track, with my mother's ashes safely returned to their container.

My brother, Antoine, whom Darette respected like a second father, escorted her to the lobby, with a few loud protests and "get-off-me's" to show her objections to being removed from the proceedings. We could hear them arguing in the lobby until he had somehow convinced her to go to the parking lot to calm down. He returned to the main seating area a few minutes later, wiping his bald head with a handkerchief, looking visibly disheveled.

"As I was saying…we don't know when it is going to be our turn next, that's all. Be thankful that God is watching over you." Josephine said quickly, and returned to her seat.

Darette came back inside and took a seat at the back of the room with her arms crossed looking totally pissed off. I had said a silent prayer of thanks that there were no cameras allowed in the funeral home that day and that no one from the media was in attendance. The gossip columnists would have had a field day with that one. I kept looking over my shoulder, though, to see if someone else was in attendance, but it looked like Duke was going to be missing in action.

It wasn't like I really wanted to see him to be with him, again. I just wanted to know what he looked like after all those years. Was he bald? Had he gained weight? Had he changed so much that I wouldn't even know what he looked like? My curiosity was getting the best of me, so I got up to go to the bathroom thinking that if he were there, maybe he would see me and catch me in the hallway before I got back to my seat.

I came out of the ladies room and stopped in the vestibule. I looked into the main seating area and surveyed the crowd carefully. The Duke I knew was nowhere to be found. But then, out of the corner of my eye I saw the figure of a large man, dressed in a long overcoat and a fedora pulled down over his eyes, lurking in the corner near the pamphlets and announcements.

He had his back turned to me and looked like he was trying to be inconspicuous. He turned slowly and lifted his head. I saw the distinguished jaw line with the graying goatee and mustache of a familiar face.

"Oh, my God, Duke...is that you?" I whispered.

"Hey, Baby...how are you doing?" The voice was distinctive.

It was definitely Duke. Although he had the paunch of a middle-aged man, the rest of his body was the same. He always wore black alligator shoes, and tailored suits, no matter what the occasion. He always looked good...*real good!* He walked toward me with his arms outstretched. We met and hugged like old friends and the years melted away when I caught a whiff of his cologne...m-m-m English Leather...just like I remembered.

"Your Mom was a wonderful woman, C.J.... We are all going to miss her terribly. You know I loved her like she was my own mother."

Suddenly, I couldn't hold back the tears any longer. The feelings of loss and grief overwhelmed me all at once and I began sobbing uncontrollably. Duke held me tightly.

"Don't worry, Baby...I'm here now. Let it all out."

Chapter 5

Fantasy

The stupid neither forgive nor forget; the naive forgive
and forget; the wise forgive but do not forget.

Thomas Szasz *The Second Sin (1973) "Personal
Conduct"*

When you walk through Hell wearing gasoline
drawers...you are going to get burned, one way or
another. For me to believe that I could actually see
Duke again without any type of repercussions, was just
plain ludicrous. I thought that twenty-five years could
erase all of the pain and lingering feelings that I might
have had for him, but they didn't and they couldn't,
especially not under those circumstances.

When we were together, Duke had spent more
time at my house talking to my mother than I did myself.
Sometimes, I would come home from working at the local

71

mall to find him there with her in our living room watching television, drinking fruit punch, and eating cheese crackers. Sometimes they would even be playing a game of Scrabble or two.

He truly loved her like she was his own mother, especially since he never really knew his own. She was "Mom" to him, and he showered her with all the love and affection he couldn't or didn't want to give to his step-mother. Mommy soaked it up like she was a proverbial sponge.

My own father had passed away a very long time ago and she had not had any male attention for well over ten years since my step-father had also died. I didn't know who my real father was until I was almost an adult, so having a loving man in my life or not, was no big deal to me. All the psycho-babble about young girls who don't have a strong male figure in their lives seeking attention from boys didn't apply to me.

I had uncles and brothers up the yin yang, who adored me, and they made sure that I towed the line as far as seeking attention from the wrong man was concerned. And then, there was Duke who protected me like my own personal pit bull. But, my mother needed attention and affection like she needed to breathe.

Duke had wheedled his way into our lives like a leech sucking on an arm for dear life. His smile could rival that of a talk show host's and he had the baritone voice of an opera singer even at a young age. Listening to him talk was like listening to "The Quiet Storm" radio program; the one whose silky-voiced announcer could make a woman swoon with imagined passions beyond her wildest dreams. He knew how to work his charms on a woman, too, no matter what her age, and Mommy was like putty in his hands. In fact, *everybody* in my family really loved him.

His personality was just that infectious. I didn't mind what he was doing, at the time, because I knew that he needed her as much as she needed him. It was innocent and very endearing in the beginning. But, when it came time for me to cut him loose, it was like pulling teeth to get him out of our home. I would tell my mother to stop letting him come into the house when I wasn't there, but she wouldn't listen to me.

"Oh, baby...he's not doing nobody any harm," she would say, trying to convince me to see things her way. "Besides...you're not here half of the time, and I need someone to cook for. All of you kids are so busy in your own lives. You don't have time for your old lady, anymore. He's good company."

"But, Mommy...I'm trying *to get rid of him*...not invite him to the wedding!

You don't understand what he is doing! Just stop opening the door!"

"But, I can't do that, baby. He's my friend, too."

It was no use trying to argue with *any* of the women in my family. We always got our way, sooner or later. We were like driven District Attorneys on the fast track to political success. We knew what to say, when to say it, how to say it, who to say it to...and, when it looked like things weren't going our way...who to *pay* to get the job done right.

My mother had worked for the local government for over twenty years and served as our county representative for two terms. Her retirement party was covered in the district newspapers. My two sisters were in show business; the oldest having started out as the manager for a struggling garage band that went on to become one of the most famous disco groups of the seventies, and the other one's husband was a well-known R&B singer who had a couple of top ten hits in the eighties. Not to mention the fact that my own career had taken off right after I had auditioned for my first gig with "The Singer".

Famous and infamous people floated in and out of our living rooms on a regular basis. We were no strangers to power and influence. Although we were not filthy rich, we knew people...people who were willing to give and return favors, if necessary.

So, when Duke became too much of a problem to my family, all it took was a phone call to the District Attorney's office and the police were at his home in a matter of days. They served him with the order of protection in person.

"What the f__k is this?" he had protested loudly from his front door.

"You just stay away from Mrs. J. or you'll be cooling your heels in a jail cell, young man," the cop had told him as he handed Duke the legal papers on the day before my wedding.

"Who asked you to do this? Mrs. J. loves me...it couldn't have been her."

"Don't you worry about who did it...you just worry about keeping your distance from that address, alright?"

"We'll just see who stays away from who dammit! Nobody tells Duke Preston what to do! My Daddy don't even tell me what to do!"

Duke had been devastated by the initial rejection. He was hardheaded and heartbroken but he wasn't stupid. Unfortunately, he also had to face reality. I had warned him that all the phone calls and presents were getting to be a bit much. But, he couldn't accept the fact that I did not want to be with him anymore. I had moved on, while he was still hopelessly stuck in the past.

I had met my fiancé, Desmond Howell, at the University of Bridgeport-Stamford in 1977 while he was studying Communications Management, and I was studying Fine Arts with a concentration in the Performing Arts. I had performed in many of the school's functions, and he was always the Master of Ceremonies with a voice like chocolate cream. Desmond and I had so much in common that it was scary. We were a match made in heaven and I thought that I had finally found true happiness.

Meanwhile, Duke was stuck back on Long Island; wallowing in the despair of having lost the only women he had ever truly loved. Every week he would try to go to my mother's house or call her on the phone. She talked to him for a little while, until one day my brother found out that he had been calling there and threatened to have him thrown in jail if he didn't stop.

They loved him, but they knew that in order for me to have a happy life, Duke had to let go of my family; a task that he dreaded and found extremely difficult to accomplish. The reality he could not accept was that you cannot make someone love you, no matter how hard you want the fairy tale to be real, --- if it is not meant to be,... *it's not going to be!*

My wedding day was a natural disaster of biblical proportions. The ceremony was my dream comes true except for the fact that a "wardrobe malfunction" had made my wedding dress totally un-wearable. My attendant had gotten the zipper of the dress stuck in the multiple folds of lace and beads in the bodice and we ended up having to literally cut me out of the dress just hours before ceremony.

I guess I had put on a few pounds with all the stress that I was going through in the months before the big day, couldn't fit into my impeccably tailored fantasy creation, and left absolutely no time for an emergency alteration to have been done. I had to get a white evening suit from one of our local dress shops as a substitute.

The disappointment on my fiancé's face, when he saw me coming down the aisle in a tacky suit instead of the $15,000 dress that his family had paid for, spoke volumes. He never did forgive me and neither did his family. They reminded me about it every chance they got. Then came the reception.

Oh my God! The reception from Hell!

We had rented a small luxury facility on the North Shore of Long Island in a sleepy little town called Glen Head. We thought that by having the reception at an exclusive place, in a remote area of town, that the chances of Duke showing up uninvited were slim to none. Little did we know that he had a few tricks up his sleeve.

First my mother had screwed up by telling him what day I was getting married in the first place. Oh, why did she have to do that? Then she screwed up *again* by telling him *where* the ceremony was going to be, thinking that I had already told him. Actually, he had used reverse psychology on her to make her think that I had told him, and that I had invited him at the last minute, but that he had lost his invitation and couldn't remember where the place was. She fell for it and then all hell broke loose!

The day of the ceremony, Duke had decided that he was going to play James Bond 007 and spy on my house. He was smart enough to keep his distance, so he got a pair of binoculars and camped out down the street and watched us coming and going from 500 yards away. He knew that he couldn't crash the ceremony in broad daylight, so he waited. He waited until everything was over at the church and then followed the limousines to the reception facility.

Then, he waited until everyone was inside and slipped in the back with the members of the entourage of the live band that my husband had hired. He managed to get a few drinks from the free bar to muster up his courage and then hid out in the men's bathroom until he heard them playing the Bride and Groom's dance song. He knew that "You are the Sunshine of My Life" was my favorite song...so, when the band started playing the first few bars that was his cue to come into the main area.

As soon as my brand new husband and I went to the dance floor, Duke rushed up from behind the bandstand and cold-cocked Desmond dead in the jaw. Desmond hit the floor with a thud. Suddenly, the band stopped playing, and everyone was in total shock because Duke had knocked him out cold!

"Get up motherf___er!" Duke had yelled. **"Get up and fight like a man, you sorry-assed P___y!"**

He continued cursing him out, while Desmond lay unconscious on the floor. He then began saying how Desmond had stolen his woman and how we had ruined his life. Then he grabbed me, and tried to plant several kisses on my lips while I fought him off for dear life. My brothers and uncles rushed him while he fought like a madman, as they literally carried him out of the building on their shoulders.

Then they held him in the parking lot, someone called 911, Desmond had him arrested, and the rest is history. Desmond spent our honeymoon in the hospital on painkillers after the oral surgeon fixed his broken jaw the next day. Needless to say, it was a rocky start to what would prove to be an even rockier life together.

As Duke comforted me in the lobby of the funeral home, I could not help but feeling a little bit guilty about how things had turned out over the years.

"I'm sorry...I shouldn't have broken down like that," I mumbled, as I wiped my face with Duke's handkerchief. "I guess I haven't really had time to grieve for my mother."

"I understand...believe me. Been there---done that, a few times. Remember?" He said with a huge smile on his face. "Why don't we get out of here and go talk somewhere?"

'Warning Will Robinson...Danger, Danger!'
As the thought kept running through my head, Duke led me toward the front door of the funeral home.

"Um...I can't leave my son alone...he needs me." I said, and turned to go back into the main seating area.

"Oh, he'll be just fine with your family," he assured me; with that confident tone he always used to get his way and then grabbed my hand. "We won't be gone long."

"Alright...but, just for a few minutes. I guess we do have some catching up to do," I conceded.

Duke and I walked towards the parking lot and into the bright sunshine of a crisp Fall afternoon. I breathed in the fresh air deeply and it revived my spirits. It felt weird walking beside him again, and the silence between us was very uncomfortable. I had to break the awkwardness of the moment.

"So...how's life been treating you? Pretty good, I hope. You look well."

"Oh you know...Life is Life...," he said.

"...and, Death is Death," we both said in unison and then started to laugh together.

"I feels good to hear you laugh again, C.J. I never thought I would ever hear your voice again. You know I bought all of your records and played them over and over again."

"I'm flattered, Duke. You know the Egyptians say that Death is Life and Life is Death ...whatever that means."

"It means that we are born again in death, and we begin to die the minute we are born again into this world," he explained.

"How did you know that? Are you still studying?"

"Of course, --- I became the shaman of a local temple right after you…you know, right after you…," he hesitated and his head dropped to his chest. I could see that he was struggling to find the words he wanted to say, so I cut him off:

"Look, Duke…we don't have to go there, if you don't want to. Let's just go back inside, and we can talk later."

"No…C.J. --- I have to get this out, right now. I've been holding it in for over twenty-five years. You know that you hurt me bad, Baby. You told me that we were going to be together forever and you reneged on me."

"I didn't *re-neg* on you…I grew up."

"The truth is that you left me…and, then you had me arrested! I know it was you who had the police come to my house to serve me with those damned papers! And, let's not even talk about the wedding reception. Life was bad for me those six months in the joint, after I was arrested.   I'm a pretty man, C.J. --- I had to fight the bullies off every day. But, I ain't mad atcha…I ain't…"

The words stuck in his throat and he looked like he was actually going to cry.

"Duke…you still don't get it, do you? I loved you, too, with all of my heart, but I couldn't take all the accusations, all the arguments, and all the insecurity. I couldn't breathe, Duke. You had me walking on eggshells the entire time we were together. I was like…you know,…that little butterfly in the poster…you had to let me go."

"But, you didn't come back…now did you?" The Bomb of Truth had been dropped.

"Oh, Look!...The service is over and the people are starting to come out.

Why don't you just come by the house later on and get something to eat?"

"Am I allowed?" he asked, sarcastically.

"OK...I deserved that one. Let's just bury the hatchet and move on, alright?"

"Whatever...it's your world and I'm just a squirrel..."

"Yeah... I know...trying to get a nut."

I knew all about it, all too well.

Chapter 6

Trickery

It is easier to forgive an enemy than to forgive a friend.

William Blake (1757 - 1827)

An hour later I was sitting in my mother's house on the living room couch talking to my middle daughter, Joanna, when we heard a slight commotion at the front door. My brother, Joaquin, ran into the living room to tell me that there was someone there to see me. I hurried to the door to find my brother Antoine yelling at Duke:

> **"You don't belong here! You need to just turn around and get the hell out of here before you cause any more trouble!"**

"I didn't come here to start anything," Duke began. He continued with his teeth clenched. "I came to pay my respects to your family and to see an old friend, you fool!"

"Don't you talk to me like that or I will cut you a new..." Antoine grabbed Duke by his lapels and Duke allowed him to enter his private space without retaliation.

I had reached the door by then and interrupted him:

"Calm down, Antoine...I asked him to come."

"Are you out of your mind, woman?" he said, and let go of Duke. "Is your memory *that short* or are you just suffering from selective amnesia?"

"I am not suffering from anything except the loss of my dear mother, and I think she would have wanted Duke to come here tonight." I said.

"Girl... Are you crazy? May I remind you, that you are a married woman? You had better watch your step...both of you!" He said, pointing his finger at us, and then he turned to go back inside to continue talking to one of his friends.

My son, Milo was behind me staring at Duke with a curious look on his face.

"Are you alright, Mommy? Who is that man?" he asked.

"Duke...I want you to meet my son, Milo Howell. Milo, this is Mr. Duke Preston. He's an old friend of mine and he might have been your Daddy."

Duke smiled at the suggestion.

"He looks like the guy in those pictures you showed us except he doesn't have all of that hair on his head, anymore."

"Good observation, young man...but your mother is still as pretty as ever, huh?" Duke remarked.

"You go on back inside, Milo…" I said, and took Duke by the arm past the living room where everyone was sitting and talking.

"You kept my pictures…?" Duke asked, quietly.

"Just a few, for old time's sake," I said, and led Duke to the kitchen where the food was spread out on a big buffet table.

"Let's just get you a plate and find a nice quiet place to talk."

I could feel the tongues wagging and the fingers pointing all over the place as we walked down the hallway. There were so many people from the community, old friends we hadn't seen in decades, neighbors and even a few strange stragglers standing all around the house and out in the yard, that I didn't think anyone besides my brothers had even noticed that Duke was there.

Aunt Jillian seemed to appear in the kitchen door out of nowhere.

"Duke Preston, ----well, I'll be damned!"

It was a miracle that she even remembered his name.

"Aunt Jillian...how are doing, Sweetheart? You look absolutely marvelous!" Duke said, while reaching to give her a hug.

She pulled away and kept her distance.

"Don't you 'sweetheart' me you...you stinking pile of horse manure!'

"Auntie!...Duke didn't come here to be insulted," I interrupted; a bit perturbed at her lack of compassion and diplomacy.

"Well, what did he come here for, then?" she asked.

"Look, Aunt Jillian...I'm just here to comfort an old friend."

"Humph! A likely story...I know your kind...been dealing with them my whole life. You wait for your opportunity and then you pounce like a snake on his prey. And, I'm not your aunt...*you can call me Mrs. Johnson!*"

"I assure you, *Mrs. Johnson*...I have only the most honorable intentions towards your niece. I am a minister now and have only come to do the work of the Lord."

"Yeah...I've heard about your little church, alright. You got them young girls over there doing God knows what for you... it ain't nothing but a sacrilegious cult if you ask me!"

"Well...nobody asked you. So, if you will excuse us," I said quickly while fixing Duke a plate of food. Then I grabbed a chicken wing for myself, and headed for the front door again with Duke close behind.

"Let's just go sit in your car and talk," I suggested. "Which one is yours?"

"The black Mercedes parked at the end of the block," Duke answered.

"You mean the big one with the gold trim?"

"Yeah...that's me. A little gift from one of my followers," he explained proudly.

Maybe my aunt had been right about him. I had been away for such a long time that I really didn't know much about what had been going on back home. My daughter had told me something about a church where the young girls were seduced into serving the minister there and providing him with all kinds of sexual favors, but she had never told me the real name of the pastor. She had told me that they called him "Big Daddy Hotep". It couldn't have been Duke...or, could it?

We reached the car and Duke pressed the automatic door opener in his pocket and the car made a "woop, woop" sound. The doors unlocked with a loud click. Duke rushed to the passenger side and opened the door for me, as I slid onto the soft tan leather bucket seats. The car smelled like it was new.

"You've done pretty well for yourself, haven't you?" I asked, admiring the freshly cleaned dashboard with the state of the art sound system, navigational board and set-in TV.

The smell of Patchouli permeated the air from the gold plated purple velvet lined crown sitting in the window. I handed Duke his plate of food and he began to eat. He didn't let me get any information out of him ,though.

"No better and no worse than any of the other preachers in town. I hope these greens weren't cooked in pork. You know I don't eat swine."

"I thought shaman preachers take a vow of poverty," I said, wondering out loud. "And, you know they cook *everything* in pork. We're from the South, remember?"

"Yeah…some of them do. But, I didn't. That kind of stuff's for priests and nuns…. I have other ways of serving the Lord. I think I'll just eat some of the potato salad then."

"Then how do you make your money?" I began to question his integrity at that point.

"Let's not talk about me. *What have you been doing* all these years, my sweet lady?"

His evasive attitude began to arouse my curiosity about him. But, I answered his question matter-of-factly. I surely didn't want him all up in my business, either.

"Well...you know...it's a long story." I said, taking another bite of my chicken wing.

"I got nothing but time...how about you?" he said, with a huge smile that made his dimples sink into his cheeks.

"Anyway...here's the condensed version: I got famous, I got married, I had three kids, got divorced, started a business, lost my business, got married again, got my business back, lost my mother...and, now I'm sitting here talking to you. Got any other questions?"

"C.J....who do you think you are talking to? This is me...Duke... 'The Man'.

Have you forgotten that I practically taught you everything you know?"

"Maybe everything *I used to know*...but, you haven't been in my life in a very long time. I've learned a few tricks of my own since 1975," I countered.

"Well, I see you still haven't learned how to keep a man with you..."

"Now what's that supposed to mean? Who the hell do you think *you are talking to?* Excuse my French, Mr. Preacher man!"

"That's not French, Darling---and I speak your language very well. If you and your husband had such a great relationship, he would be right here taking you out of this car. So, where is he, anyway, C.J.?"

"That's none of your business...and we are doing just fine, thank you very much! We have some issues to work out, that's all...like any other married couple."

His interrogation struck a raw cord in my being. I was trying desperately to hide my disappointment from someone who connected with me on a more ethereal level than any other man I had ever met in my entire life.

"All I know is that if you were *my wife*...I wouldn't let you out of my sight!"

"Well, then, speaking of wives...where is *yours?*"

"We broke up a *long* time ago. I've been single for over ten years. We got married in 1979, had two children...a boy who's twenty-four years old now, just graduated from college with his MBA, and a girl who's twenty-one years old,... graduates next year with her pre-law degree. We had some... religious differences...and she didn't agree with the direction that I was taking my church... so she left me. I haven't spoken to her in over two years since my son's graduation. I don't date much. The church pretty much takes up all of my time and energies. I don't need anything else in my life... except maybe a good woman who understands me like you do."

He leaned in closer to me and tried to lay his head on my shoulder.

"Duke...I'm a married woman, and I don't intend to...to...to," I hesitated to finish my sentence and lifted his head off my arm.

"And, neither do I...," he began, "...intend to try to force you to do *anything* you don't want to do. I'm just here for you to cry on my shoulder if that is what you need, Sister C.J."

"I don't need you or anyone else to tell me how to live my life. I am doing just fine, thank you very much and don't need your damned shoulder to cry on anymore, either." I grabbed the handle of the door and started to jump out of the car.

"Have it your way, Sister C.J.. You have my number. Don't hesitate to use it if you need to. My 'office' is open 24/7."

"I doubt if I'll be needing anything from the likes of you! And, I'm not your sister!"

I got out of the car, and slammed the door behind me.

"Hey…take it easy! That's a sixty-thousand dollar door you're slamming there!" Duke yelled out of his open car window, then he started the engine and took off down the street.

I watched as the car turned the corner and moved quickly out of sight. I glanced at my rented van parked in the driveway and sighed heavily. Marcella met me at the front door as I climbed the stairs.

"I told you he was going to be trouble," she said.

"He's no trouble…I know how to handle his kind." I said confidently, and slowly walked back inside the house.

That night as I lay in bed watching TV in my old bedroom, my cell phone rang at 12:00 am. The caller I.D. told me that it was Sly. It was getting late and I was hoping that he hadn't forgotten about me.

"Hi, honey…!" At first I was happy to hear his voice.

"Hey, baby! How are you doing? How was the funeral?" He asked.

"Oh…you know. It was rough on all of us."

"You sent everyone my love, didn't you?"

"Yeah…but they all wanted to know why you weren't here, though. How was your trip?"

"Well…you know how much I hate to fly. But, once we got up in the air it wasn't too bad. It was the landing part that freaked me out, though." He chuckled, lightly.

"Tell me about it! What goes up must come down, huh?"

"Yeah, right! ---- You miss me?"

"Like a flower misses the rain…"

"You keeping it tight for me?"

"What's that supposed to mean?" The question raised my curiosity.

"I just miss you that's all…you know I can't fall asleep without you holding me."

"Oh yeah… I'm just a little wiped out that's all. I was fighting sleep waiting for you to call me. Can I call you back in the morning, Hon?"

"Sure but, wait, C.J.….I just wanted to tell you that I love you, baby. Every thing's gonna be alright."

"I love you, too, Sly…Smooches!"

"Alright now,---Behave yourself."

"Of course, I will… you, too. Bye."

I hung up the phone and an uneasy feeling washed over me. Sly hadn't been that loving and sweet to me in weeks. My woman's intuition kicked in and I decided to call him back. Five minutes later I called his number again and his answering service picked up. I didn't leave a message. Five minutes later I called again. This time he answered.

"Shut up, y'all! Hello...? Hello, are you there? Hello?"

As he spoke I could hear music, laughter and muffled female voices in the background. I kept silent and just listened. Suddenly the music cut off and the voices stopped.

"Hello?--- C.J.? Is that you?"

I hung up the phone without saying a word. Then, I went into the bathroom to take a sleeping pill. My phone rang again, but I decided to not answer it, and twenty minutes later I was knocked out. He never did call back.

Chapter 7

Infirmary

If you do not wish to be prone to anger, do not feed the habit; give it nothing which may tend to its increase.

Epictetus (55 AD - 135 AD)

The pain in my solar plexus shook me from my sleep early the next morning. I stumbled to the bathroom to put cold water on my face. Everyone else in the house was asleep, or so I thought. I was praying that no one had heard me moaning and groaning as I sat on the toilet, trying to compose myself. My daughter Joanna walked into the room and sat on my bed looking very worried. She waited until I came out of the bathroom to speak.

"Mommy...are you alright?"

"Um…I'm fine, baby. It's just a little gas. You know, ---all that rich food we were eating yesterday."

"I don't think gas can make you moan *like that.* Are you sure that's all it is?"

"Of course, I'm sure. Now you go on back to sleep or doing whatever it was you were doing. What *are* you doing up so early, anyway?"

"Shawn called and he wants me to come back to school right away. He just said that his roommate and his roommate's girlfriend had a fight over some girl and they had some trouble with the police. They got kicked out of the apartment where they were living and he needs someplace to stay. He wants me to let him stay in my room at the dorm until they find another place. They have to be out of their apartment by tomorrow morning."

"Oh, Lord…what is wrong with you children? Everything with you all is violence, sex and problems. Now you know I don't approve of you living with no boys."

"Mommy…it's not like we are celibate, you know."

"I don't want to hear about it! I also don't want to hear that you have been kicked out of the dorm for having unauthorized guests. So you do what you gotta do, but you make sure *he* gets his own place right away. A man doesn't respect a woman he has to lean on for his support."

"Well, isn't that what Sly is doing with you?"

I never hit my children when they were little because I did not believe in corporal punishment, but that time I couldn't control myself. The slap sent Joanna reeling over the side of the bed onto the floor. She screamed in pain and started crying as she balled up into the fetal position. I ran to her side immediately.

"Oh my, God! Joanna! I am so sorry, baby! Oh my, God! What have I done?"

"Get off of me! Get off of me! Don't touch me! Get away from me!"

She slid across the rug on her behind and struggled to get up.

"Please let me help you, Honey…I didn't mean to hit you like that. It's just that…you know, I've been under so much pressure, lately. I just…I just don't want you to make the same mistakes that I've made in my life. You can understand that, can't you?"

"No! I can't understand anything you do! What kind of mother hurts her children like this? We never see you …you're always on the road…you never come to see me at school…all you do is send me money. You don't even know what's going on in my life! Do you even care?"

"Of course I care, Honey! What kind of monster do you think I am anyway? Come on now…Let me help you up. Here, here…sit down over here."

We sat down on the side of the bed. I gave her a big hug, and wiped her face with a tissue. Her big sister came into the room with Darice close behind.

"What's going on, Nammy? --- Why is Auntie Jo Jo's face all red like that?"

My inquisitive granddaughter couldn't help asking the obvious.

"We just had a little accident that's all… everything is alright now. Right, Joanna?" Joanna was silent.

Before anyone could say another word, the pains in my solar plexus struck again and made me double over. I fell into Marcella's arms.

"Mommy!," she screamed. "Mommy, what's the matter? Are you alright?"

"Call …911…" I said, and fainted.

I awoke two hours later on a gurney in the emergency room of Southside Hospital. My daughter, Marcella, was standing over me, holding my hand. I was feeling very groggy from the painkillers the doctors had given me.

"What happened?" I asked her,

"We don't know...you tell me. Joanna said you told her you were having gas pains, then you two had an argument, you slapped her, and the next thing we knew you were passed out on the floor. I never knew that a fart could kill you."

"Right...Neither did I. What did the doctors say?"

"They're doing some tests right now and we're waiting for the results. You were delirious with pain. Don't you remember?"

"I don't remember anything, except...Where's Joanna?"

"She took the train back to Philly. She said to call her and let her know what's going on later. She's really mad at you. She said you hit her for no reason."

"It's Shawn…he wants to move in with her," I said.

"I know…she told me all about it. So, let them do their thing."

"Their thing could cost me a lot of money. And, I'm not going to let her mess up her life, like…" I stopped short and Marcella finished my sentence for me.

"Like what? Like I did, Mommy?"

"No…now you know I would never say anything like that, Marcella."

"But, you *thought it,* didn't you? Look, I had Darice because I couldn't stand being in that house with you arguing with Des, and all of his stinking girlfriends anymore. Where were you,

Mommy? I needed a mother in my life not a disco queen; running all over the world. You didn't even tell me about you and Lenny until I was almost thirteen years old! Don't make the same mistakes with her that you did with me, Mommy. Joanna has always been your Golden Child, but she's not as perfect as you think she is. She's flunking out of her first semester. Did you know that?"

"No...I haven't gotten her grades in the mail yet."

"Well, she is...and, she said that she's thinking of dropping out of college and doing some other things to make money."

"What other things?"

"You know...like stripping, maybe...selling crack cocaine."

"Oh my God...now you're trying to kill me!"

The doctor came down the hallway with a clipboard in his hand. He stopped next to the gurney and introduced himself. He was friendly and soft-spoken.

"Hello, ladies...my name is Dr. Kirkpatrick, and I am your attending physician. It appears you had a bit of a problem this morning, huh?"

"Yes...So, can you tell us what's wrong with her?" Marcella asked.

"Well...Mrs. Greene...it looks like we need to do some more tests. I can't give you a quick prognosis right now. But, we will know in a few days exactly what is going on. In the meanwhile, we'd like to admit you for a few days and..."

"Woa..woa...woa...pump your brakes, Doc! I can't stay in the hospital. I have to get back to Atlanta."

"Mrs. Greene...you're not going anywhere in your condition any time soon. If I release you, I would be signing your death warrant and you may never make it back to Atlanta. I suggest you relax and settle in for a long winter's nap, young lady."

"Oh, my God...did you call, Sly, Marcella?"

"Yeah...I left a message on his cell phone. He hasn't called me back yet, though."

"It's just five o'clock in the morning in California... he isn't even awake yet. He usually sleeps until 12:00, anyway. Try again in a couple of hours. Or, just keep trying until he answers."

"Uncle 'Toine said he was coming out here as soon as he can. He said traffic on the Long Island Expressway is horrible this time of day, so he's gonna wait until nine o'clock, if you're not dead by then. Everybody else went to work."

"Great...Thanks a lot, baby. I'll just lay here and make my peace with the Lord 'cause I'm gonna be dead one way or the other as soon as we get the bill from the hospital for this."

"O.K. then, --- I'll just go sign the papers and get you checked into your room. What kind of insurance y'all got?"

Insurance? Did I pay my insurance bill that month? Oh, Lord...I didn't even know if I had the right health insurance coverage or not! Milo was being covered under his father's insurance according to the custody agreement, Joanna was being covered under her school's insurance, and Sly was still being covered under his last employer's policy. I had just sent away the health insurance packet for my business and didn't even know if all the paperwork had been processed or not.

"I can't even think about all that right now," I answered.

"Well you'd better think about something, because they asked me already, and I told them that I didn't know. They said that they needed to know before noon." Marcella reminded me about the hospital's policies for new admissions.

"Otherwise, they're gonna transfer you to County General in Nassau, and you never know what kind of treatment you're bound to get over there!"

"They're not going to transfer me anywhere. I said I'll take care of it."

"Well, alrighty then..." she said as she walked briskly towards the nurse's station.

A few minutes later a familiar hand touched my shoulder as I snoozed on the gurney.

"C. J., --- I'm here." It was Duke.

"Oh my God, Duke...what are you doing here? How did you know I was here?"

"I have a police scanner in my office. I can listen in on 911 calls and I recognized the address when they answered the call from your mother's house. I kept my old C.B. scanner to keep tabs on my followers just in case of an emergency. And, this looks like an emergency to me," he explained.

"Why did you come here? I was so rude to you yesterday. I didn't think you'd ever want to see me again."

"C.J. you keep forgetting…this is old Duke. I know everything about you that I need to know. I know you didn't mean what you said to me, and I know you need my shoulder to cry on again, now don't you?"

"Duke, come on…give me a break, O.K.? I'm a big girl now. How did you get in here, anyway?"

"I just told them that I was your husband. They asked me about the insurance coverage and I told them to just send the bill to the church."

"Where's Marcella? I thought she was taking care of all that."

"I saw her outside on the phone talking to someone. Meanwhile, I know that you can't afford to pay the hospital, because, they also told me that they were going to transfer you to County General if someone didn't given them the proper insurance information today."

"Look, Duke…I'm not a charity case. I don't need your help and I don't need your money, either!"

"Apparently, you do…"

The silence in the room was deafening.

"And, I will pay you back every penny just as soon as I get out of here," I said, finally.

"Don't you mean *if* you get out of here?"

"Oh, I'm going home, alright…" I said, and tried to get off the gurney when another pain knocked me off of my feet.

"You aren't going anywhere…and neither am I. I will stay right here as long as you need me to." Duke said, as he helped me to get back under the covers and then sat down at the foot of the gurney.

"No...you'd better get out of here," I said, panting and out of breath. "My brother, ---Antoine is coming."

"Alright, I'll go...but, I won't be far away. Here's my card, Baby. You call me when you get your phone connected. Remember... 24/7 just like I said."

He kissed me on the forehead and the aroma of English Leather filled my nose, again. He turned and I watched his muscular silhouette glide down the hallway towards the exit; his black alligator shoes clicking on the linoleum floors like the sound of tiny rhythmic drums. Something primal stirred within my being; something that had been dead for a very long time. I licked my lips and laid my head back on the pillow to take a nap.

Chapter 8

Yes, Regretfully

There is nothing like returning to a place that remains unchanged to find the ways in which you yourself have been altered.

Nelson Mandela(1918 -2013), *'A Long Walk to Freedom'*

I lay in that hospital bed staring at the ceiling contemplating my life. Had I been a good wife and mother? Had I done everything in my power to make my husbands and my children happy? Had I really been as selfish and uncaring as Joanna said I had been? I had gone through so much in my life, and put them through so much, that I may have shut down emotionally, and not allowed myself to feel their pain because I was so afraid to feel my own.

Happiness in my eyes was having a roof over my head, food in my stomach, nice clothing to wear, the love of adoring fans, and a man who worshiped the ground that I walked on. Being loved was extremely important to me; almost as important as having a million dollars in the bank. I would have sold my soul to the devil to have a man in my life that could provide all of those things without making me feel unappreciated.

An ungrateful man is the vilest creature to ever walk the face of the earth in my eyes. But, had my search for the perfect mate, preceded the needs of my children and my family? Could I have been so selfish as to forget about what they needed first?

My first marriage had been a shambles from day one. We were too young, too inexperienced, and too stupid to know any better. We thought that money ruled the world and that having a large bank account could cure every problem we would ever face in our lives together. Desmond had come from an extremely wealthy Jamaican family and never knew the struggles of poverty.

I had come from an upper-middle class family and worked my way to the top of the heap through hard work and talent. Money or the lack thereof, was never an issue in our lives. But, money is not the solution to everyone's problems

I thought we were happy because I assumed that Desmond understood my need for love and attention. (We all know what happens when you ass-ume something, right?) He had his own stellar career as a D.J. for one of the most popular radio stations on the East coast by the age of twenty-four. His name was as well-known as my own. We commanded the best tables at the most popular clubs, and we had the world on a string.

Our first few years together were simply heaven. And, then reality hit us smack in the face. I should have known that his fragile ego could not stand being upstage by a woman...not even his own wife.

Desmond had wanted a family in the worst way, but we hadn't planned on what the obligations of taking care of children would do to our personal lives together.

Also we were on different time tables. Desmond was no more than an emotional child himself and I had some serious emotional issues of my own. He had demanded that his career come first because he was the MAN! And, although I was a "liberated" woman, he only allowed me to be liberated in public.

Behind closed doors he was as chauvinistic as they came. He knew that one day my popularity and the demand for my services would wane. He knew that the music business was a cruel mistress who demanded so much more than her lovers could provide. And, he took advantage of that knowledge in the cruelest ways possible.

After three exciting years of touring with "The Singer," I was finally offered a record deal of my own in 1981. I was ecstatic and came home one night after a gig to tell Desmond the good news. He was less than impressed.

"You're not *that* talented, C.J....you'd be better off in the background with the other girls."

"I thought you'd be happy for me. What is your problem, Des?"

"I thought we were going to start a family this year," he had protested, assuming that I was in total agreement with him; but it was something that we had never really discussed fully in detail.

"Well that's going to have to wait a minute," I had said. "This is my dream come true, Des, why can't you support me in this? Why does everything have to be about you?"

"This is not about me, C.J.---it's about our family. Remember 'family'?...The reason why two people get married in the first place...to be together and make babies? Didn't you say you wanted two kids and a big house in Connecticut?"

"We can still make babies, Des…just not right now. And, we already got the big house…so we're halfway there, right?" I had said, while giving him a big hug and a kiss; trying to get on his good side.

I believed that he would accept the plans that I presented to him. I would cut my first album, go on tour for a couple of years, make some money *and then*, start my family. I had been on the road for a fairly long time, and most of it was during the first part of our marriage. So, thought that he had gotten used to my being away, and wouldn't mind a few more years of my traveling around the country.

Unfortunately, it didn't work out that way, *exactly*. Six months into the tour, the album was nominated for a Grammy for best new female artist and I was walking on cloud nine for weeks after the nominations had been announced. I had been home on a two week break and was preparing for the trip to California; constantly talking about how exciting it would be if I actually won.

Desmond and I had made love that week like two teenagers on prom night. I was finally feeling satisfied, beautiful and fulfilled, all at the same time. Little did I know that all was not what it seemed to be.

The day of the taping of the ceremony, we had tickets to catch a flight to Los Angeles from La Guardia airport in Queens, NY. We were supposed to have had lunch in the city and then drive to the airport for our trip. But, Desmond had been in a bad mood that whole day and seemed to be disturbed about something.

I found out later that his bosses had threatened to cut his hours or put him on the overnight shift because his ratings had dipped a little in prime time and he was not a happy camper. When it came time for us to leave he announced at the last minute that he wasn't going with me. He said that he hadn't been feeling well all week and I, being the understanding one, accepted his excuse to stay home.

Although I was extremely disappointed that he couldn't be there with me, I was more excited that I was going to meet some of my favorite artists and that I was finally going to get the recognition that I had always dreamed. To make it even more exciting, my agent had told me that I had seats *right behind* Patti La Belle, *and I could not wait* to get the chance to talk to her!

I flew to Los Angeles with my manager, Lenny, and kept in touch with Desmond back home right up until just before the ceremony began. He claimed that he would be going to bed early that night and that he would wait for my call as soon as the winner was announced. Well, unfortunately…I didn't win.

But, I was thankful for the nomination because it meant that the sales of my record would skyrocket and that people who had never heard of me would finally be listening to my music. I called Desmond to give him the news and got a busy signal for over two hours.

I tried again later on but, the after-party and all the photo shoots kept me occupied and pretty well distracted the whole night. Lenny served as my escort for the evening and the night passed quickly. Everyone in the industry knew that Desmond was my husband, and they soon began to question his absence. My explanation about his illness raised some people's suspicions about our marriage being on the rocks.

It seems that Desmond had been seen at another industry party in New York with an assistant from the radio station, about three months prior while I was out on the road, and rumors of a breakup had begun to circulate. Lenny was understanding and supportive, but he also had his own agenda that night, and expressed his opinions about Desmond to me later on at the after-party.

> "Desmond, couldn't give a crap about your career or your real _happiness, C.J. ...There are some things you don't know about your loving husband!"

> "What are you talking about, Len?"

"He's seeing another woman whether you believe it or not."

"Well, I don't believe it. You're just jealous of our relationship!"

"Well...you had better wake up and smell the coffee, Lady. Because you seem to be the only one who doesn't know about it, C.J.. Look, --- *I'm the one* who cares about you. *I'm the one* who has been by your side all these years, watching you develop and grow into one of the most talented singers I have ever represented in my entire career. I want to be the one that you come home to after a long stretch on the road, not him. I want *you* to be happy so *we* can be happy together!"

Lenny grabbed me by the hand and we walked arm-in-arm to one of the rooms in the hotel that the club had reserved for their private parties. He closed the door behind us and pulled a joint out of his breast pocket. We shared a passionate kiss and I sat down on the bed to catch my breath. He walked to the mini-bar and pulled out a bottle of champagne.

"Here is to your nomination, C.J....you will always be a winner in my eyes."

He popped the cork on the champagne, lit the joint from a candle that was burning on the table and came to where I was sitting on the bed. He blew the smoke from the joint into my mouth and I inhaled deeply. We drank champagne, and made love until the sun came up. But, as we got ready to catch our plane the next day, I realized that we had made a big mistake. I did not love Lenny like I loved my husband. But, the damage had already been done and it was too late to turn back.

The next day, I had finally managed to reach Desmond on the phone around noon.

"Hi, Baby...Are you feeling better, now? What happened? Why didn't you pick up the phone last night? I wanted to give you the good news."

"Oh...I'm so sorry. I must have knocked it off the hook when I reached for my medicine last night. I went to bed about nine o'clock and slept like a baby."

I found out later that he had spent the night with his assistant-girlfriend.

"Well...I didn't win. But, I got the chance to talk to Patti *and* Lionel Ritchie! I said excitedly. "Lionel was a little stand offish, but Patti was very down to earth. She gave me some advice and autographed my program. We had *a really good time!* Everybody asked about you."

"Good...I'm glad you had a good time. I don't mean to cut you off, Sweetheart, but, I have to go take care of some business at the station."

"Oh...alright, Baby. I'll see you when I get home. My plane gets in at about eight o'clock Eastern Time...I'll take a limo from the airport straight home and I'll see you later."

Men lie because *they think* that women are stupid and will forget what they have said to them. Women lie because *they know* that men are stupid and *will* forget what they have said to them. I lied whenever it was convenient for me to get my point across. My plane actually got in at six o'clock and I'd wanted to surprise him to have a little late dinner with him.

I told the limo driver to take me straight to the station on the East Side. Traffic was heavy but we made it there in about forty-five minutes. I knew that he took dinner at seven o'clock when they were changing D.J.'s, so I gave myself ample time to make it there.

We pulled up to the front of the station, drove into the parking garage and before I could even get out of the limo, I saw Desmond and his eighteen year old assistant coming out of the lobby arm in arm. They passed right by the limousine, laughing and talking. They even stopped to smooch a little right before getting into his car and driving away. I was devastated and shocked.

I told the limo driver to follow the car, which he did. Desmond drove a short ways across town to a sports bar, where the two of them went inside for approximately an hour. At eight o'clock on the nose they came out, got into his car and drove away. I didn't need any more proof. I told the limo driver to take me straight home to Connecticut.

We lived just a short half-hour drive from the city in Bridgeport. He arrived home shortly after nine o'clock, almost nine-thirty. I was waiting in the bedroom. He came up the stairs and called out my name.

"Yo...C.J....where are you? You home yet?"

I met him at the doorway of the bedroom in my sexiest negligee, with my hair flowing down my back, my makeup done perfectly, looking my very best. I wanted to know how much he missed me and I acted like nothing was the matter...just like he did.

"Hi, Baby...where have you been? Did you miss me?" I said, in my sweetest, sexiest voice.

"What do you mean? Where have I been? I've been at work all day and just came home to be with my wonderful wife. Did I miss you? Of course, I missed you! Damn you look good! Come here girl!"

He started kissing me on my neck and moved his way down to my breasts. My passions stirred, I couldn't hold back and I let him take me right there on the floor of the bedroom. After all, I had been away for a while and missed my husband. I wasn't going to miss the *best "breakup" sex* I had ever had in my entire life. Besides, I wanted him to see what he was going to be missing very soon.

After we finished, I broke the news to him nonchalantly.

"Guess who I saw today, Des?"

Then, I told him the whole story about how I came home early and went to the radio station to meet him. I told him all about who I saw him with, where they went, and what they did together. I told him about the rumors of him being with this girl for months. He was in shock and he actually *tried to lie his way out of it,* but I wasn't hearing it. I had witnesses and proof. The next day I went downtown to the courthouse to file for a divorce. I didn't tell him about me and Lenny, though, and I kept *that* little secret to myself.

Unfortunately, Fate had a different plan for us. Two weeks later, I found out that I was pregnant. It seems that with all of the excitement of the Grammy's, I had forgotten to take a couple of my birth control pills.

We got back together a few weeks later, I forgot all about the affair with the assistant, and our first daughter Marcella was born later on that year. I put my career on hold and became the consummate housewife and mother…for a little while at least.

But, I was not made for motherhood and housework. I was not used to being home; fooling around in the garden or shopping at the Mall on Saturdays. As soon as our daughter was old enough to walk, I got back into rehearsals and hit the road again.

I hired a nanny and left all of the mothering chores to her. Desmond had not entirely mended his cheating ways, though. His affairs with other women lasted on and off for another five years. He even had sex with our nanny!

I was so busy performing and making a name for myself that I didn't care, anymore. Lenny and I got closer, but our relationship remained purely platonic. He was my knight in shining armor and my protector on the road, but he was just my close friend and confidant. Since, he looked so much like Desmond, we never thought to question who the father of my first child was. It was a secret that remained hidden until many, many years later.

My marriage was a total shambles at this point, and several times I had secret sexual affairs with either members of my band or an industry big shot to seal a record deal, or even a choice groupie or two. Drugs and alcohol were plentiful and there was always the opportunity for me to get the attention I wasn't getting from Desmond at home, from the men that I was around on the road.

Every concert tour ended in a party at some fancy hotel, and every awards show meant that I would be out of town away from the tensions created by my husband, and available for fun and games to make me forget my troubles. Lenny would try to stop me, but basically he just made sure I didn't get killed by a jealous girlfriend or by the drug crazed fans that followed us around.

I got pregnant again late in 1987, and decided that I was going to settle down and finally put my singing career to bed. It wasn't until early in 1992 that I had had it with all of the touring and life on the road. Fifteen years of living out of a suitcase and ten years of arguing with Des about our family and his philandering, not to mention my own brief affairs, had taken its toll on my nerves and I needed a rest. I had to spend three months in a rehab center for cocaine and sleeping pills addiction while dodging the paparazzi and the media gossip magazines.

My middle daughter, Joanna was about four years old by then, and after I retired, I had gained over forty pounds from just laying around the house watching soap operas all day. Desmond would make snide remarks about my weight and he started watching porno videos just to get aroused for sex. Our relationship took a nosedive for the ultimate worse.

Marcella was almost twelve years old, when she started looking and acting more and more like her real father, Lenny. One night after one of our infamous arguments about nothing in particular, I finally got up the nerve to tell Desmond and Marcella what had happened the night of the Grammy nominations and after a paternity test confirmed the facts, it was the nail that sealed the coffin on our dead marriage.

Desmond and I stopped sleeping in the same bed. We stopped living in the same bedroom. We lived like brother and sister and only had sex once a month out of obligation when both of us were horny at the same time, but there was no more love between us. Marcella stopped talking to me because she was angry that I had not told her who her real father was sooner.

Five years of therapy had absolutely no effect on our relationship. Our problems were much too deep, and the fact that both of us were no longer bringing in as much money as we used to make made the arguments even worse. **It had always been about the money.** Our financial obligations were huge, and my taste for the finer things in life was unbridled.

I had married him thinking that he was a responsible, caring and wonderful man, when he was nothing more than a selfish, emotionally stunted child. We realized that we had never really loved one another and separated for almost two years. Desmond moved into an apartment in New York City with his girlfriend and I stayed in Connecticut in our home. He visited the children on the weekends like all the other part-time fathers and we stayed married in name only. Our life together was in marriage limbo hell for over two years.

During that time, I had started my own designing business. It was just sort of a hobby at first and I never took it seriously. But, I discovered that I had a talent for decorating and after taking a few classes at the local community college, I took on a few clients. Desmond and I reconciled for a short time, he moved back home, and I got pregnant again in 1994 with our son Milo.

But, we were far from being happy together. Desmond was just not satisfied with his life. He was getting older and the young chicks weren't digging him as much as they used to. His heyday on the radio was over and I had ballooned up to two hundred pounds during the pregnancy. He became bitter and mean.

One night he came home in a very nasty mood. I was cooking a snack in the kitchen. He came into the room and threw his keys on the counter.

"I want a divorce...woman."

"What do you mean...you want a divorce? I thought we were working things out for the kids?"

"I talked to my lawyer and he suggested that *you* move out since this house is *my family's* heir property and I want to sell it."

"Heir property, my ass...*this* is *my home*! Where am I supposed to go, Des?"

I was pissed.

"Well...like Rhett told Scarlett...frankly I don't give a damn!"

"What about the kids, Des? You're kicking *your kids* into the street? What about their schooling and their friends?"

"I'm filing for custody of the kids. They're staying here with me. And, I don't care what you do with your bastard daughter."

"You cold-assed motherf____ker...I hate you!" I flew from behind the counter and attacked him right there on the spot.

We went at it like two WWF wrestlers in the ring. He tried to twist my arm and I kicked him in the groin. He fell to the floor and I grabbed a knife from off the kitchen counter.

"You take my kids from me and I will kill you! You bastard!"

"You kill me and they won't have a mother or a father…is that what you want?" he had said, lying on the floor gasping for breath and holding his genitals.

"I'm not leaving this house, Des. Wild elephants couldn't pull me up out of here!"

"Maybe not wild elephants…but this restraining order can." He pulled the paperwork out of his lapel pocket and threw it up on the counter. "After I call the police, and they see these scars… your ass will be going to jail for the night!"

I never knew that I could feel that kind of anger and hatred for a human being. I grabbed my coat and my purse and ran out the door. I could hardly see where I was going from the tears in my eyes.

"Make sure you have your stuff out of my house by tomorrow!!" I could hear him saying, as I hopped into my car and took off down the street.

I didn't even know where I was going. It was after ten o'clock at night and it would be after midnight before I could get to any of my relatives' houses. On the side of the highway I saw a Motel 6 in the distance. I pulled into the parking lot in front of the management office and sat in the car for a few minutes to compose myself.

I booked myself for three days, not knowing what I was going to do or how I was going to handle the fact that my soon-to-be ex-husband had just totally devastated me and was trying to ruin my life. I cried myself to sleep that night.

The ensuing events could fill volumes. The custody and divorce proceedings were a virtual nightmare that took over two years to complete. He claimed that I was an unfit mother and couldn't take care of my children because I didn't have a "real" job and was technically homeless. He stopped payments on the car I was driving and had it repossessed. I had to start driving one of my older vehicles instead.

He canceled all my credit cards that were in his name. He tried to drag my name through the mud and brought up a past misdemeanor drug arrest that I had acquired when I was a teenager in college. He let them know about my time in the rehab center. In the end, the judge gave him temporary custody of the kids claiming that he could provide a more stabile home for them than I could.

I had to put all my stuff into storage, move back to my mother's house with Marcella, and sleep on her living room couch because the house was full of other relatives. I traveled back and forth to Connecticut by train and taxis to see my other children, who asked me when

Marcella and I were coming back home every time I saw them.

My heart broke to pieces each time we saw them, and they cried and begged me to not leave every time that I had to go back to Long Island. Marcella was beginning middle school and started becoming a disciplinary problem. She would get into fist fights with the other girls in the neighborhood and I had to go to her school almost every week for conferences with the assistant principal. The stress of it all made my hair fall out in clumps. I lost my budding business and all of my clients.

I lived off of what little savings I did have, and found a part-time job at a fabric store in the Mall. I had to give my employer my real name and he remembered me from when I worked there during my college vacations. I told people who thought they recognized me that I was mistaken for the famous singer they knew and loved, all the time.

I had to cut what little hair I had left off and start wearing a wig. I gained another thirty pounds and was celibate for two years; not being able to bring myself to trust men again. My only consolation came when I started to go to church and became a born-again Christian. I studied the Bible nightly, got baptized, prayed that God would work things out for me in my life, and that I would finally get my children back. When the trial was finally over, I had regained custody of the children, *lost forty pounds,* planned to move to Atlanta, and the rest is history.

Desmond lost his radio job in 1998. He moved out of his family's house to go live in California, and the last thing I heard, was that he was working part-time for a local apartment complex as the Superintendent. He designs websites in his spare time and hangs out on the beach watching the pretty girls go by all day. He's lost all of his hair and put on about fifty or sixty pounds.

Revenge really is a bitch.

We only speak occasionally to talk about the children. I know that he is not happy, but his happiness is no longer my concern. We never apologized for any of the hurt and pain that we put each other through over the years. I guess that getting away from him was "sweet relief" to me, after all was said and done.

Antoine came into the room and interrupted my reverie.

"Yo, Sis!...How you doing?

He leaned down to give me a kiss. I turned and wiped the tears from my eyes and off my face. I was still groggy from the medicines the doctor had given me.

" Oh, hey...'Toine. 'Toine, do you think...I'm a good mother?"

"Now what's brought this on? What are you talking about?"

"I had a fight with Joanna, and she told me that I was a bad mother. Do you think I am, too?"

"C.J....you've been through a lot with those deadbeats that you married. You need to think about getting well right now."

"Deadbeats? Sly is *not* a deadbeat! He's a good man, and he's been very good to me."

"Oh yeah? Then, where the hell is he?" The question hurt my feelings badly.

"You know he's in California...He can't just jump on a plane and get here like that!" I snapped my fingers.

"I would...if you were *my wife*."

"He doesn't even know that I'm in the hospital, yet," I said, while adjusting the covers on the bed nervously.

"We've been calling him since this morning, C.J.. He hasn't even answered his messages. Look, Sis...you just think about getting better, right now.--- Alright? Now...do you need anything?"

"As a matter of fact, I do need *something.*" I hesitated for a few seconds; searching for the right words to say. "I need someone *else* to take care of my hospital bill for me and to lend me about two thousand dollars."

"Someone else...what do you mean 'someone else'? Who's taking care of it right now, and why can't they *just keep right on taking care of it?* And, what's the two thousand dollars for?" he asked.

"Duke Preston wants to pay for everything...but I can't afford to pay him back right now, and I don't want that kind of favor hanging over my head. I need to cover some late bills until one of my clients pays me. I'm waiting until my health insurance to kick in to pay the hospital, and this trip is costing me a fortune. Can you cover me?"

"Sis...now you know I had to take care of *all* the final expenses for Mommy, pay for Stacy's tuition last month and the business is not doing so well right now...it's the slow season."

"What am I going to do, then?" I was desperate at this point.

"I'd let old Dukey-boy pay... I think he owes you for messing up your wedding day like he did and I wouldn't worry about paying him back. I might be able to front you a few hundred in cash to tide you over for a couple of days, but that's about it. So, how come Sly can't? Oh, I forgot...he's living off your money. I'm sorry, Sis...but it's the truth, ain't it?"

"We *share* our money!! He makes good money, too. We just have a temporary cash flow problem, that's all," I explained.

"Well...here's two hundred...and I'll see what we can do about the other stuff later." He reached into his pocket and pulled out a roll of bills and peeled off two.

"Don't worry about the kids, they're just fine. Marcella is taking care of everything. She said she'll be back a little later on, and that she had some business to take care of. Right now you need to rest."

He kissed me on the cheek again and waved goodbye. I watched him walk away wishing that we could have completed the money transaction. I hesitated for a few seconds and then reached for my purse sitting on the night table. I put the two crisp one hundred dollar bills into my wallet and caught site of the business card that Duke had given to me. I pulled it out and looked at it for a minute and then picked up the telephone. I got a dial tone and dialed the number on the card. A very youthful sounding female voice answered the phone.

"Hello...Temple of Everlasting Faith...may I help you?"

"Hello...may I speak to Duke Preston, please?"

"Oh you mean, Father Hotep? Hold on please."

It was true! Duke was the preacher of the church where the young girls were being seduced, just like my Aunt had said he was. I hung up the phone without waiting for him to answer. A few seconds later the phone rang. I hesitated to answer it and let it ring a few times. After the third ring I picked it up.

"Hello...?"

"Hello, C.J....What happened? Why didn't you wait for me to pick up your call?"

"Um...I...didn't want to disturb you, *Father Hotep,*" I said, sarcastically.

"Well, then...why did you call me? And, you know *you* can still call me Duke."

"Duke,...I...just wanted to...um, ...thank you ... for offering to pay my hospital bill...I don't know how I can ever repay you, though."

"Oh...that's not important. I think we can work something out. I'll be there in a little while to talk about it."

I started to feel a little uneasy about the whole situation, but felt like I was definitely stuck **"between a rock and a very hard place"**.

Chapter 9

Slippery

Seize the moment of excited curiosity on any subject to solve your doubts; for if you let it pass, the desire may never return, and you may remain in ignorance.

William Wirt (1772 - 1834)

Duke rode down the highway in his big beautiful car, with a huge smile on his face, thinking that he had finally accomplished the one thing he thought that he could never do again in his life...get me back. He had me just where he wanted me, under his obligation and in his good graces. Little did he know that God was still in control of his flock and still in control of my life.

As he pulled onto the expressway, he got a call on his cell phone.

"Hello...Father Hotep, here...what is your desire?"

"Father Hotep...this is Leticia. We have an emergency at the church. The F.B.I. are here to question you about something. What do you want me to tell them?"

"Tell them that I am out of town and won't be back until the end of the week. Stall them for me until I can figure out what to do. I'm a go to my Dad's house in Holbrook for a couple of days and you hold it down for me, alright?"

"But, Father Hotep...I can't...I can't..." she said, excitedly.

"Leticia...*yes. you can do this!* And, when I get back you and I will go on a little trip together, alright? How does Jamaica sound to you?"

"O-o-o Big Daddy...that sounds niiiiice!"

"Right....You just tell the other girls to lock up the books and hide all the computer discs in the basement vault. Lock up all the doors and, I'll see you in a couple of days, OK?"

"Alright...Big Daddy! I'll be right here waiting for you."

"Oh Leticia...you know are my special girl. And, don't you ever forget it."

"I won't, Big Daddy Hotep! I'm your faithful servant, forever."

"Good, girl...I'll see you later."

Oh, he was smooth.---- As smooth and slick as a greased up python, slithering through a vat of Crisco. The girls who worked for him were all no older than twenty-five. All sizes, shapes and all colors. As soon as they reached their twenty-fifth birthdays they had to leave their positions in the office and move to the general population. The general population was basically all young people between the ages of sixteen and thirty who were either "run-aways" or "throw-aways" from their biological families.

Father Hotep preached a philosophy of freedom from the shackles of society's rules. He taught his followers that rules and laws were made by the leaders to control the minds of the masses. He led them to believe that if they followed him, that they could achieve all the desires of their hearts…if they would only give up their attachments to money and things, by donating everything they owned, and 50% of what they earned to the church.

He dressed up in these long purple robes during his sermons and burned a particularly strong brand of incense to add to the atmosphere of mystery and secrecy. Candles were placed in the pulpit and throughout the small room where he held his "learning sessions", as he called them. He taught them about using the powers of their minds, to achieve greatness and to acquire power over their enemies who, naturally, were their parents, their teachers (if they were in school) and anyone else who objected to what Father Hotep was telling them.

They all lived in this big old house with about seven bedrooms in it, across the street from the church. They were sworn to secrecy and not allowed to leave the house without permission from Father Hotep. Although he swore that his followers lived there voluntarily, the contract that they signed upon becoming a member said otherwise. The penalty for disloyalty to the church was total banishment.

In this case, banishment meant being taken, while blindfolded, to a remote area of upstate New York in a darkened van, and dropped off without food, money, clothing or any way to communicate with the outside world. Having heard the rumors about one of the disloyal followers having been eaten alive by a black bear while trying to find their way out of the mountains, was enough to keep the others in line.

What he did with the young girls was the worst exploitation one could imagine. Duke took full advantage of their worship of him. He made them feel like he was Jesus incarnate, and that he had some special powers over them, especially in bed, which he would share with either one or two of them at a time. They actually would fight over which one was going to be the special chosen ones for the night. He had them wrapped around his little finger like little bees going for the mother lode of honey.

He would tell them that their sexual power was natural gift from God and that they should be free to express themselves in that way without restraint. Some of his philosophies were good, but he mixed them with the vilest forms of mind control that anyone could ever experience. He performed rituals in the basement of the church, using dead animals, and a form of drug that was mixed up in the kitchen using medicinal and hallucinogenic herbs.

The girls were deprived of food and sleep for days, and he would punish them by locking them in their rooms for days at time, if necessary, until they promised to behave, totally. He would make them have sex with one another so he could watch them get off. They had no idea what he was doing to their minds or their bodies. Many of the girls got pregnant.

One of the girls' parents had decided that they were going to rescue their daughter from his clutches. They had not seen or heard from her in over two years and had heard that she had become a member of Father Hotep's church. So one night, the mother who looked rather young for her age, falsely petitioned to become a member of the church at one of their open membership ceremonies. She was taken to one of the back rooms to be prepared for her initiation. One of the assistants was her own daughter.

"Chandra...it's me, Mommy!" she said to her daughter when she was finally alone in the room with her. "I'm taking you back home."

"Mommy?...I have no mother," her daughter answered. "Father Hotep is our mother and our father. Father Hotep is the 'All in All" and this is my family, here."

"Chandra...snap out of it! Now, come on, now... I'm getting you out of here." She grabbed her daughter and pushed her towards the door.

But, I don't want to leave! Let me go!!!" Chandra had screamed and pulled away from her mother.

But, before anyone realized what was going on, the mother had grabbed her daughter tightly and rushed out the back door where her husband was waiting for her in their car. That was how the community found out what was going on in the big house on the hill. The young girl who was rescued, eventually recovered and told the local newspapers all about Father Hotep's practices.

However, as long as the girls were there voluntarily, which is what they had told the police when they came to investigate, no one could ever pin anything on Father Hotep. He made sure that they were "of age" or close to it before he introduced them to his filthy ways. He thought that he was invincible.

From that day on, large body guards watched over every move those girls made. Father Hotep paid his guards well and there was never a shortage of young men, mostly former crack heads and drug dealers who wanted to change their lives, who came to the church for a place to live and a free meal. They sold books, and jewelry and all kinds of trinkets to make money for the church.

Some of the children came from very wealthy families, who paid large sums of money to get their children away from the clutches of Father Hotep. He would tell the police that the ransom/bribes were donations to the temple. This was the man to whom I now owed a huge debt. I hadn't the slightest idea how I was going to pay him back, nor how I was going to explain to my husband how or why he was back in our lives.

I lay in that hospital bed thinking about the bills and the loan, and little beads of sweat began to pour off my forehead when the doctor came into the room with his trusty clipboard in his hand.

"Mrs. Greene...I'm glad you're here alone. You look a little flushed, let me get a nurse in here to take your temperature and your blood pressure. You don't look, too well."

"I'm alright, doctor...I just have a lot on my mind right now."

"I can understand that, Mrs. Greene," he began as he listened to my heart with his stethoscope. "I take it you've been under a lot of pressure lately. Mmmm-hmmm---just as I suspected."

"What do you mean...'just as you suspected'? What do you suspect? What's wrong with me?"

"Mrs. Greene you are suffering from an acute case of neurological fatigue and severe peptic stress ulcers. You have heart palpitations, an unusually high blood pressure, you're overweight, and you are at risk for a sudden stroke. We caught it just in time. If you don't get some rest and have an operation to relieve the pressure of the ulcers on your solar plexus, and get your blood pressure down...well, to put it frankly...you will die!"

"Die? Oh, my Lord! ....Jesus save me!"

"Now take it easy, Mrs. Greene. You're not going to die right away. In fact, you're not going to die at all, because we are going to take very good care of you and you are going to leave here feeling 100% better in a couple of weeks."

"A couple of weeks...? Doctor Kirkpatrick, I have a business...I have a family...I can't spend weeks in a hospital."

"Well then, have it your way. Either, you spend a couple of weeks here letting us doing what we need to do for you, or we can invite you to come back here in a body bag. It's your choice."

Marcella walked into the room and stood behind the doctor.

"What's your choice, Mommy? What did he tell you?"

"Doctor, can I be alone with my daughter for a few minutes?"

"Of course, Mrs. Greene. Your mother is a very sick lady," he said to Marcella. "Please, tell her to do the right thing," he said bluntly, turned, and left the room.

"What did he say, Mommy? What's wrong with you?"

"Nothing that a big bottle of E & J and a week in Jamaica wouldn't cure." I said, jokingly, and then told her everything that the doctor had just told me about my condition.

As the doctor walked back to his office, one of his colleagues who was also working on my case, stopped him in the hallway.

"Doctor, I saw you coming out of Mrs. Greene's room, have you told her the bad news?"

"Yes, I told her as much as I wanted her to know right now," Dr. Kirkpatrick told him.

"It's a damn shame...this AIDS epidemic is really getting out of hand," said the colleague.

"Yes, I know...we'll deal with that bombshell later. She has enough on her plate to deal with right now."

Chapter 10

Ecstatically

If we had no winter, the spring would not be so pleasant:

if we did not sometimes taste of adversity, prosperity

would not be so welcome.

Anne Bradstreet *'Meditations Divine and Moral,'*
American poet (1612 - 1672)

Marcella sat on the bed holding my hand for what seemed to be an eternity. She was my best friend and really the only person to whom I could turn in my time of need since my mother had died. Now that Mommy was gone, Marcella was my rock.

"Did Sly call you back?"

"Not yet, it's still pretty early in Cali..."

"Keep trying, Baby...he probably forgot to turn his phone on again." I reminded her.

"Mommy...what are you going to do?"

"What do you mean...what am I going to do? I'm going to lie here, get well, and let the chips fall where they may. And, speaking of chips...I'm starving. I missed breakfast, can you go get me something from the vending machine? They won't be serving lunch for another hour or so, and I am famished."

"Sure, Mommy....I'll see what I can find. What do you want?"

"Something natural...and healthy," I told her. "Get a granola bar, and some ginger ale."

"O.K...I'll be right back," Marcella said, and walked off down the hallway in search of my snack.

My TV was tuned to the morning newscast. I turned my attention to the screen for few seconds.

"...And, all of the winners of the largest Lotto jackpot in the history of New Jersey since the games began have yet to come forward to claim their prizes. The six winners will each share a jackpot of over thirty million dollars with the cash option. That's thirty million dollars each, folks! I could certainly use some of that money! The winning numbers again were: 6, 26, 32, 37, 45 and the Mega Ball number was 51. Congratulations to the winners! I am sure there are some very happy people out there this morning. And, now in sports... the Knicks had an impressive win at the Garden last night..."

'Why did those numbers sound familiar?' I thought to myself. 'I must be dreaming or doped up on painkillers, especially if he said that the Knicks won last night.' I grabbed my purse out of the nightstand and searched for the little pink ticket in my wallet. It was still folded up between the gas receipt and the change from the coffee I had purchased in Jersey. I could only remember about three of the numbers, but when I unfolded the ticket I almost fainted. I had at least three of the numbers the announcer had called out. Two more and I could claim a prize of at least $250,000. Three more and I was set for the rest of my life!

Just then, Marcella came back into the room.

"Baby...Baby...Go get me a newspaper!"

"You couldn't have asked for that when I went out the first time?" she complained.

"Just go get the newspaper, girl, and I'll explain to you why later."

"Oh, alright..." she said, while stomping her feet.

She threw the snacks on the bed and went back out to find the paper. A few seconds later my cell phone rang in my bag and I reached in to answer it. The caller ID told me that it was Sly. I almost didn't answer it.

"Hello...?"

"C.J....Baby...how you doing?"

"What do you mean...how you doing? Have you listened to your messages, yet? Why haven't you answered your phone?"

"Oh, damn! I must have left it on vibrate last night! I see now someone tried to call me. I didn't recognize the number, so I didn't think it was that important."

"I'm in the hospital you knucklehead!" I said, angrily.

"The hospital? What the hell are you doing in the hospital? What happened? Did you have an accident or something? Are you alright?" he asked, excitedly.

"No...I'm *not* alright. I'm stressed out, I got an ulcer and some other stuff is wrong with me. The doctor said I have to stay in here for two weeks or

else I might die! Sly, I need you with me, baby!
How soon can you get here?"

"Oh, man...I don't know, Sweetheart. I'm right in
the middle of these negotiations here. We're
meeting with the money people tomorrow, and I
can't just up and leave right now," he explained.

I started to get irritated.

"You are my husband...you are supposed to be by
my side! I need you to be here, Sly! I'm your wife.
I am supposed to be the most important thing in
your life. Where are your priorities?"

"My priorities are for me to take care of business,
so I can *take care of my wife*, so she can *stop
taking care of me,* so I can be a *real man* to her for
a change! But, then you wouldn't know anything
about dealing with a *real man*, now would you?
Because, you won't let me be a real man!"

Marcella walked back in the room with the
newspaper tucked under her arm.

"Look...I can't talk about this right now... you know they don't allow cell phones in the hospital. The doctor said that I have to stay as calm as possible and get my rest. I'll talk to you later."

I disconnected the call and lay my head back on the pillow. The phone rang again. It was Sly.

"I said I can't talk right now..."

"C. J., I'll be there as soon as I can, alright? I love you, baby."

"Whatever..." I said and hung up the phone.

"Was that Sly?" Marcella asked.

"Yes...and he can't get here right away. He has a meeting with the business people and he can't get a flight out of Cali until later on in the week."

"I swear...I don't even know why you married that loser."

"You wouldn't understand...," I said softy, and closed my eyes.

"Here's your paper. What's so important, you need to read about it right now?"

"Oh shoot...I almost forgot!"

I grabbed the paper and looked for the Lotto numbers on the first page. I compared the numbers in the paper with the numbers on my ticket. I had just two more numbers for a total of five. I hadn't won the jackpot, but I was a second place winner of $250,000!

"Oh my God, Marcella...I won! I won second place...I'm a winner!!"

"What are you talking about? Give me that..." Marcella grabbed the newspaper and the ticket and looked at the numbers. "Oh, my God, Mommy...we're rich! All our troubles are over!" she said and started dancing around the room.

"*Our* troubles? What 'choo talking 'bout, Willis?
I know *my troubles*, or at least some of them are over. *You* need to go buy *your own* Lotto ticket, Girl."

"Oh, Mommy...you're cold."

"I'm just joking! Oh, Marcella,--- this is the answer to all of my prayers! I can take care of the hospital bill, pay off all my other bills *and* take a vacation! Virgin Islands here I come!"

I thought for second...I had to keep this a secret! I couldn't let too many people know about my fortune. I would have relatives crawling out of the woodwork all over the place.

"We have to keep this a secret...Marcella, you can't tell *anyone* about this."

"Not even the family?" she asked.

"I said *nobody*...and *especially* not the kids...and especially not anyone in the family. I'll break the news to them later. Right now I am going to lay here and plan my vacation. You just tell them that I'm feeling *much, much better* and that I will be home soon. Give Milo the phone number here and let him call me. I'll talk to Sly myself. I'll call

Joanna tomorrow, and we'll work out our difference later."

Marcella agreed to keep my secret and she left. I felt another pain starting to come back in my abdomen, but it soon subsided. I don't know if I was doped up on at the medicine or if I was on a natural high after finding out about the money. It would be another thirty days before I got a check so I had to plan my moves carefully. I broke open my granola bar, popped the ginger ale can and pretended that I was drinking champagne and eating caviar on a white sandy beach in the Virgin Islands.

Chapter 11

Vulnerability

What I am actually saying is that we need to be willing
to let our intuition guide us, and then be willing to follow
that guidance directly and fearlessly.

Shakti Gawain 1947 - present

I slept better that night than I had slept in the
last five years. The next morning the nurse came in to
take my temperature and a blood sample and told me
that they had heard me snoring loudly that night. I
apologized for making such a racket and they said that
they understood that I needed the rest. Three days
passed and I felt better and stronger than I had felt in
twenty years.

Joanna and I made up, and Sly arranged for a
flight out of California to arrive that Friday. The only
person I told about the money was my brother Antoine,
and I told him that I had just won the three number

prize of $5000. I also told him that I couldn't pay him back right away, but he understood and gave me a month to give him the two hundred dollars that he had just lent to me. The car rental company gave me a waiver for three days, since it was not my fault that I had became hospitalized and the insurance covered the extra charges.

My client finally brought the check for the full amount they owed me to my office in Atlanta and my assistant deposited it into the company bank account. The bank gave me the extension I needed to pay for my car, I paid all the overdue charges, and I arranged to get my Mercedes back. The only thing I needed to do was to take care of the money that I owed Duke.

That Thursday evening he showed up at the hospital with a huge bouquet of flowers for me.

"Oh, my God...Duke, you really didn't have to do this. Thank You."

"No trouble, sweet Lady. Nothing is too good for my C.J."

His compliment and assumption that I wanted to have anything to do with him disturbed me. But, I couldn't let him know that I didn't need his dirty money any longer right away. I had another three weeks to go before I could pay him back anything. He continued:

"You are looking a whole lot better these days, I must say."

"Well, thank you for the compliment. I am feeling a whole lot better, too. But, um...what have you been doing these past few days? I kind of expected you to visit me everyday like you said that you would. What happened?"

"Oh, yeah...I had some important church business to take care of that took me out of town for a few days. He acted nonchalantly. "As a matter of fact, I have to leave town again for a few more days this weekend. But, um...I'll be back on Monday, bright and early to see my old buddy."

The truth of the matter was that the F.B.I. was investigating attempted murder and molestation charges that one of his followers had filed against him, and the I.R.S. was investigating his income and bank accounts. The story was all over the news and Duke was trying to keep a low profile. My curiosity took over.

"Duke...um...Why are they saying those things about you in the newspapers? Is it true what they say about your followers and how you treat them?"

"My followers are grown people who have minds of their own. They don't need me to tell them what to do or not to do," was his retort.

"But, what about the money, Duke? "

"I make my money just like any other preacher. I get donations, tithes and offerings. It is all very legitimate." he explained, very matter-of-factly.

"And, what about the young girls...you know,... um...," I hesitated to talk about the sexual aspect of his teachings fearing that he might get angry and he would be offended.

"What about the young girls? I only deal with grown women who are serving their community. What they desire to do with their bodies is their own business. I don't force anyone to do anything."

He was starting to get agitated, so I decided to change the subject.

"You know…um, the doctors have told me that I might be going home sooner than they thought. My blood pressure has stabilized and the medicine that they gave me for the ulcers has practically healed them completely. I can't thank you enough for all the help you have given me."

I should have gotten an Academy Award for that line.

The thought of having to rely on that snake in the grass for another minute actually made me ill inside. But, I had to maintain my cool until an alternative plan presented itself. I had to get well fast and get out of that hospital bed before another penny of charges had been added to my bill.

"I'm very happy for you, Miss C.J."

"Oh now...don't you be so formal...you know that you can call me, C.J." I raised my arms to give him a hug.

As he leaned down to hug me, I saw the figure of a man behind him. It looked like my husband.

"Sly? ---Oh my God,...it is you!" Duke stood up and turned around quickly.

"What the hell is going on here?" Sly asked, calmly.

"Um, Sylvester Greene, this is an old friend of mine Mr. Duke Preston. Duke this is my husband, Sylvester."

They politely shook hands. "Nice to meet you..." they said simultaneously, without a hint of emotion from either of them.

"Oh man, --- I am so glad to see you, Baby! Come here!" I said, reaching out to hug my husband.

He brushed past Duke, came to the bedside and allowed me to hug him tightly. I almost pulled him on top of me in my exuberance. I really wanted Duke to believe that we were a happy couple.

"What are you doing here so early, you sly devil, you?" Sly stood up and looked straight at Duke.

"Well now, you know…I managed to take care of my business early in California and now I'm here to take care of business with my wife."

"And, your wife and I have a little unfinished business of our own to take care of" Duke added, with a smirk on his face.

"What's he talking about, C.J.?" Sly asked. I could almost see the hair beginning to stand up on the back of his neck.

"Um,…well, …um, Duke here …was generous enough to help me get my hospital bill straightened out. He is…he is…the pastor of a local church … uh …a temple actually,… and if it wasn't for him I would probably still be lying over there at County General, in the emergency ward doubled over in pain… Ha, ha, ha!" I chuckled, lightly.

"Yeah…ha, ha, ha…" Sly repeated, sarcastically. "Well, I am here now. So thank you very much, Mr. Pastor…whatever-your-name-is."

"That's Father Hotep, to you," Duke cut in.

"Father Hotep? ---Now, why does that name sound familiar?" Sly asked with a puzzled look on his face. I tried to run interference before he got too suspicious.

"Um…Duke was just leaving…weren't you Duke?"

"Yeah…I got some business to take care of myself."

"Well it was so nice seeing you again, Duke. ---
And, I'll be talking to you soon about that hospital
bill, O.K.? You take it easy." I said, smiling
broadly; trying to get him out of the room as soon
as possible before Sly started asking him any more
questions.

"Nice talking to you, too, *Mr. Greene*...You have *a
very lovely wife*, there. I'm quite sure the two of
you are very happy. You have a nice day." Duke
said, as he tipped his hat politely and turned to
leave.

Sly sat down in the chair with a puzzled look on
his face.

"Why did you need him to take care of your
hospital bill? I thought you got insurance through
your business."

"It's a long story, Honey. You know how those
health insurance policies are so complicated. Let's
not worry about all that now. I'm so glad to see
you! Sit down and tell me all about California!"

Sylvester sat down in the chair next to my bed and told me all about how he had met with the limousine company executives and that he and his friend, Steve, were going to do a joint venture to provide limos for the Grammy's, the American Music Awards, the Golden Globes *and* the Oscars. I was so happy that my husband was finally achieving some of the goals that he had set for himself and that we would soon have some extra money in the bank. But, there were still some lingering doubts in my mind about that telephone call I had made the night before I landed in the hospital.

"Sly…what happened the night of the funeral last Sunday? "

"What do you mean?" he said, trying to act all innocent.

"You know exactly what I am talking about. Don't try to play coy with me. I called you and I heard female voices and loud music. What was going on…a little party?"

"Oh you know...the fellas...," he chuckled. "...they had some of their women over and we had some beers, watched some videos, ate some food... but, that's all."

"Some videos? What kind of videos?"

"You know...some bootleg stuff. Bad sound... horrible resolution...the usual."

"And that's all?"

"That's all...C.J. Stop nagging me about it! You know you are the only woman in my life. I love you baby." He got up to come to the bed and give me a hug. "Being so far away from you just makes me realize how much I miss being *with you*." He leaned down again to give me a kiss.

God...I missed my husband. If I didn't think that someone could walk into the room I would have nailed him right then and there.

"So...what's going on? What did the doctor tell you?" he asked.

I repeated the whole boring prognosis the doctors had given me, and explained the procedures they were going to do to relieve the pressure on my ulcers. Sly wasn't exactly the most technical kind of person, and didn't really understand everything that I had told him, but he did understand that I loved him and that I needed to rest.

I couldn't bring myself to tell him about the money though, because, I knew that he would have tried to convince me to spend it on his business venture, and I wasn't too sure I wanted to do that right away. I had other plans for that money. My business came first.

"I'm going to go talk to the doctor and I'll be right back," he said. "What's his name again?"

"Dr. Kirkpatrick...his office is on the third floor. You should see his name on the door."

"O.K., I'll be right back..." he said quickly, and went to go find the doctor.

Dr. Kirkpatrick and his colleague, Dr. Maney, were sitting in their office discussing their patient files. Sly knocked on the door, apologized for interrupting their conversation and introduced himself.

"Oh, no trouble…Mr. Greene. We were just about to come down to the room to talk to your wife."

The doctor looked like he had something very important to tell us. "Mr. Greene, your wife's condition is very serious. She's made remarkable progress in the last week but she is far from being out of the woods, just yet."

"What do you mean, doc?" Sly asked. "Let's just cut to the chase, alright?"

"Mr. Greene have you ever had an HIV test?"

"HIV test? What's this got to do with HIV? You mean AIDS?"

"Your wife tested positive for HIV, Mr. Greene---and we suggest that you get tested also…and, very soon, I might add."

Sylvester dropped down into the chair at the side of the doctor's desk and almost lost his breakfast right there on the floor of the doctor's office. He loosened his collar and took off his hat. If he wasn't such a dark-skinned man, he probably would have turned a few shades lighter.

"We also suggest that you wait to tell her, because she is not strong enough yet, to withstand the news right now. We are telling you this for your own benefit to give you the opportunity to do what you need to do for your own health. In the meanwhile, we must keep this a secret. The news could give your wife a stroke or even worse…a heart attack. If you love your wife you will keep quiet until she is stronger," Dr. Maney cautioned him.

"Whoa, whoa, whoa...Just let me think about this for a minute," Sly said, nervously.

"Take all the time you need," Dr. Maney added. "Would you like a glass of water?"

"Yes, please..." and after a few seconds Sly said, nervously: "I can't go back into that room. I can't do this. Tell my wife I had an emergency call and had to leave. I'll see her later tonight. I have to go get some air."

"Sure, Mr. Greene...we understand. We'll take care of everything." Dr. Kirkpatrick helped Sly get to his feet. He took a few seconds to compose himself, then, he slowly walked dazed and stunned down the hallway back to the parking lot.

The doctors continued their conversation.

"It's a shame we had to break it to him like that," said Dr. Maney. "I'll go talk to Mrs. Greene, now."

Chapter 12

Secretly

There is no remedy for love but to love more.

Henry David Thoreau (1817 - 1862),

Three days later, on Sunday morning, the doctor told me that I had healed enough for them to finally discharge me from the hospital. Sly had been right there by my side from the day that he got there (except for those few hours after he got the bad news) right up until the doctors gave me the news that I could go home. He would come visit me in the morning, stay until lunchtime, and then leave for a few hours. He would come back again in the evening to have dinner and watch a little television.

The three day stay gave him time to visit my family and get to know my other children better. He tried his best to keep the secret about my health from me, but I could tell, every time that he was there, that something was on his mind. He would sit in that chair next to my bed and stare at the TV, then turn his head and look out the window for a minute like he was concentrating on something. I finally asked him what was going on.

"Oh, you know...I'm missing a lot of income being here with you. I'm just a little worried about catching up, that's all."

"Sly...I don't think we need to worry about losing money, or paying our bills anymore."

"What are you talking about, C.J.? How much money did you get from that preacher man, anyway?"

"I didn't get any money from him. He's just taking care of the hospital bill, and I'm gonna pay him back just as soon as my health insurance kicks in. I think I can get them to back date the bill so I can submit it to the insurance company. But, that's not what I am talking about."

"Well, what are you talking about?"

His curiosity was starting to get the best of him, and, I wanted to tell him about the Lotto ticket so bad that I could scream it at the top of my lungs to the world, but I had to hold back. I couldn't tell him the news just yet.

> "Um...I spoke to the girls at my company and they told me that...um...we just got a big job from a very prestigious client in Alpharetta, and they want me to redo their whole mansion from top to bottom. It's a $50,000 job, so I think we will take it. And, you're gonna be making a lot more money with the job in California, so we're not going to have any more problems paying our bills, right?"

I had to think of something to explain the increase in our bank account when I deposited the first check from the Lotto commission in three weeks. I still wasn't sure I wanted to tell him about my winning the whole $250,000. I didn't want him to control *that much* of *my* money.

"C.J. ...I'm going to be away for a very long time and I'm just not sure about how this deal is going to pan out with Steve. He's not the greatest business man in the world and I'm just worried about leaving you alone in Atlanta, that's all."

"Oh...I think I'll be just fine. You go on to California and do your thing, Baby. I'll be alright."

Just then Dr. Kirkpatrick came into the room.

"Mr. and Mrs. Greene--- How are you doing, today?"

"We're just fine, thank you." I answered.

"I'm glad to hear that. Now that you have made such a fine improvement, I think we can talk about your continued care when you leave the hospital."

Sylvester shifted in his seat, coughed a little and started to look a little worried. The doctor continued.

"First...let's talk about your diet."

"Oh...my family is vegetarian and we eat very healthy foods, thank you, " I began to tell him.

"Well, you must be doing something wrong... because you're cholesterol was way too high and your blood pressure was, too. What was your diet like before you came in here?"

"Oh you know...the usual." I looked really guilty at that point. "I may have cheated a little..."

"Um, hum..." the doctor looked at me over his glasses.

"OK...OK...I was eating a lot of fried foods, skipping meals, and I had a bacon, egg, and cheese sandwich with home fries, grits and butter every morning *and* I washed it all down with sweet ice tea and E&J at night."

"Bacon...and E & J, huh? Well, Mrs. Greene, you are fifty pounds overweight, your sodium and cholesterol levels were through the roof, and you need to really get serious about eating regular meals. Regular, healthy meals like salads, fruits, whole grains, oatmeal to lower your cholesterol, and lean meats like broiled chicken instead of chicken fried steaks and gravy.

That stuff will literally kill you, as you can see. You have to cut out the liquor and the sugary drinks and drink more water---eight glasses a day. If we hadn't caught your condition when we did, you might not have made it back to Atlanta. You could have had a stroke on the highway and killed yourself and your family."

"I know doctor...I promise to change my ways."

"And, you too...Mr. Greene. I see you could use some trips to the salad bar instead of the sports bar!"

"I hear ya, doc," Sylvester added.

"Now I suggest that the two of you work out a diet and exercise plan that works for the both of you, and we will see you back here in, let's say, 30 days for a follow up, or we can schedule a follow-up appointment with one of our affiliates in Atlanta. You need extensive continuous care to monitor these levels in your body."

"We will work something out," I said speaking for my husband and myself, while Sylvester nodded in agreement from his chair by the window.

"Alright...I will send the nutritionist in this afternoon and she can work out some menus with you, and I guess I will start working on your discharge papers. You take it easy and I will be seeing you later."

Suddenly, Sly jumped up and caught the doctor by his arm as he was leaving the room.

"Hey Doc...can I talk to you for a minute?"

The two of them went into the hallway and I could hear them speaking in whispers and low tones.

"Doc...what about the...you know...the HIV?" he asked.

"Mr. Greene...I cannot tell your wife about her status at this point. I want her to get stronger. In the meanwhile, the two of you need to have a serious discussion about your future together. You are going to have to figure out how this happened. That is not my business. My business is making sure you don't pass this horrible disease on to anyone else. I suggest you get tested, like I told you to, and once your status is determined, we can take it from there. One day at a time," the doctor advised him.

"You're right, doc. One day at a time," Sly agreed.

He turned to come back into my room and the doctor walked down the hall to go back to his office. Sylvester sat down at the foot of my bed and looked at me with the most curious look on his face that I had ever seen. He actually looked a little pale.

"What's the matter, Hon? What were you talking to the doctor about?"

"C.J. ...Do you love me?"

"What do you mean...do I love you? Of course, I love you! I married you, didn't I?"

"That's not what I mean. I mean, do you love me, enough to forgive me if I didn't tell you the truth?"

"You mean if you out-and-out lied to me? Or, do you mean if you just didn't tell me the whole truth? There's a difference."

"Well...what's the difference?" he asked.

"The difference is...a lie is when someone asks you a direct question and you deny that something has happened. Not telling the whole truth means you just left something out, while you were telling part of the truth. Now, which one are you talking about?"

"I guess I mean the one about not telling the whole truth," he answered.

"What do you mean, Sly? What are you talking about?"

"I'm talking about what happened the other night out in California. I have to know, how much do you love me, C.J.? Do you love me enough to stay with me even if I f___ked up?"

"Oh, God, Sly…what did you do? Did you sleep with someone?"

I've never had a man come to me and out-and-out confess his infidelity to me. I've always had to find out from finding a phone number, or hearing it from other people, or catching him in the act. The mere fact that he was coming forward, and being a real man, to *tell me* that he had a moment of weakness touched me.

Statistics have shown that almost 60% of men have cheated on their wives. Almost 40% of wives have cheated on their husbands. 50% of first marriages end in divorce. Only 30% of those divorces are due to infidelity. The other 70% of the marriages that are dissolved are due to money problems, illness, abuse or some other cause.

The statistics clearly show that the infidelity rate is much higher than the divorce rate, thus there are a whole lot of people out there who are screwing around, but at the same time, someone else is forgiving them and their marriages are remaining strong.

Statistics also support the fact that there are far more women in the world than there are men. So, what are all the single women in the world supposed to do for love and affection? I need a real, human being to give me attention and maybe take me out on the town every once and a while; not a drawer full of battery operated toys.

I don't fault a man for having more than one woman in his life, as long as he is honest about the whole situation, and everyone involved is aware of what is going on. That way, the participants can make their own decisions about whether or not they wish to be involved.

There is no deception, no betrayal, and above all no hurt feelings or violence.

You may not agree with my philosophies, however, I decided a very long time ago, that if my husband ever came to me and told me that he was cheating on me, that I would not have a knee-jerk reaction to the revelation. After what I went through with my first divorce, I decided that I would take into consideration all the factors that led up to the infidelity, decide whether or not I would be better off with or without him, *and then* decide whether or not I wanted to get a divorce.

Apparently, a lot of other women, ---*especially those whose husbands are in show business or sports*, have made the same decisions. Sometimes it is better to try to work things out rather than just go for the jugular vein and call the divorce lawyer.

"I didn't sleep with anyone...but, it's not as simple as that." He confessed.

"I had sex with someone for about five minutes at my partner's house."

"Sly…what the hell is wrong with you? Why are you telling me this now? Haven't I been through enough this week, now I have to deal with this crap?"

"C.J.….I love you so much. You don't understand. It's hard for men to say 'no'.

I mean, one minute we were there watching porno movies, and drinking beer, somebody pulled out a blunt, and the next thing we knew those girls were taking off their clothes and the rest of the night was kind of a blur…"

"A blur, huh?   A blur…I thought you said it lasted five minutes. And, I thought you said you were watching bootleg movies!!" I was livid.

"Yeah, a five minute blur…I stopped her in the middle of what she was doing to me, jumped up and spent the rest of the night out in my car. I would never disrespect you like that."

"Why couldn't you just leave before it got to that point?"

"I ain't no punk, C.J....the other guys were doing it, and I didn't want to look like no p----y-whipped, faggot. I got my pride, woman!"

"You didn't want to look like a faggot, so you decided to desecrate our marriage vows. Oh that's rich, Sly!"

"C.J., have I ever mistreated you? Have I ever hit you? Have I ever brought another woman up in your face? I've worked hard and I've helped pay the bills every month. I'm a good man, C.J., and I love you with all my heart and soul. Please believe me, baby. God I love you!"

He broke down and started crying like a baby on my stomach.

"I love you, too, Sly...At least *I think* I still do." His reaction seemed extreme for the situation.

The next day we left early in the morning to go back to Atlanta.

Chapter 13

Panicky

Wealth is the parent of luxury and indolence, and poverty of meanness and viciousness, and both of discontent.

Plato (427 BC - 347 BC), *The Republic*

How do you live a lie and keep a secret all at the same time? The truth of the matter was that I loved my husband but I wasn't "in love" with my husband. I was still "in love" with Duke after all these years, but he turned out to be the kind of person that I didn't want to have in my life. But, how do you explain that to someone who just confessed one of the worst things he could ever confess to a woman he claims to love?

I married Sylvester because I thought that I would never find another man to love me. I was in my late forties and I bought into the statistics that said that a woman over forty had a better chance of getting hit by lightning, while wearing asbestos drawers, standing in a lead box on top of the Empire State Building on a sunny day--- then she did to get married. He said he loved me. He wanted to get married and I believed him.

When you've spent the last five years of your life either being celibate or going on the worst blind dates you have ever had in your life,--- you jump at the chance to be with someone who at least has all his teeth, doesn't do drugs, isn't addicted to Internet porn, and hasn't spent the last ten years of his life in jail. Sylvester might not have been my best choice, but he certainly wasn't my worst either. At least he was sincere.

I wanted a successful marriage like I wanted to be a size eight again, and I took my wedding vows seriously. This time it was going to be for the long haul. This time it was going to be until death did part us and not a twenty-something year old "hoochie-mama" in a mini dress. When Sly confessed that he had had a moment of weakness, I believed him, I forgave him, and we moved on with our lives. That is what mature people who love one another do.

We made love, as usual. We ate breakfast in the morning, as usual. We continued trusting one another, as usual. Nothing had changed in our lives except the fact that we had learned that we were human beings capable of moments of strength and moments of weakness. Our world was about to be shattered by something a little bit more serious than infidelity.

Three weeks later, Sly was in California working with his partner. They were doing well, he was sending me money regularly, and he had promised me that he would make sure that he would not allow himself to get into any compromising positions that he could not handle. But, that other bombshell was about to be dropped. The check finally arrived from the Lotto commission.

I held it in my hand and stared at the number of zero's in the amount. It was real! My financial prayers had been answered. But, I had to tell the media that I could not allow them to photograph me, nor could they publish my name in the paper. They complied with my wishes and I deposited the check into my company account. I was on my way! I went to my purse, took out the business card from Duke, and dialed the number excitedly.

> *"The number you have reached _____is not a working number. Please check the number and dial again or ask the operator for assistance."*

'Well, I'll be damned'...I thought to myself. "I wonder what happened."

Then I dialed the number again and got the same recording. Then I dialed my daughter Marcella's number. She picked up right away.

"Hello...Marcella? "

"Hi, Mommy...how are you feeling?"

"I'm doing just fine, baby. Marcella, do you know what happened to Duke's church?"

"Oh, Mommy...where have you been? Oh, I forgot...You don't know what happened do you? The FBI came up in there, raided that place *and shut it down!* The IRS found out that he hadn't paid taxes on all that money he was taking in in over ten years! He owed over a million dollars in back taxes and was accused of child abuse, sexual harassment and child molestation."

"Oh, my God! What happened to Duke?"

"They hogtied his ass and carried him out of there kicking and screaming like a little girl, ---that punk! I told you he was no good. I guess the news hasn't reached Atlanta yet. Go on the Internet and look it up and see for yourself."

"Yeah...I'll do that. How's everybody else doing?"

"Everybody is good. Listen--- I gotta go, Mom. My client just walked in."

"O.K. baby...I'll talk to you later."

I hung up the phone in total shock and went to my computer. I logged on to the New York Newsday's web page and did a search for "The Temple of Everlasting Faith". Duke's picture popped up on my monitor. He was shackled from his waist down; being led away from the church by a couple of burly police officers.

The headline read:

"Temple Preacher Convicted of Molestation and Tax Evasion Charges Scheduled to Serve 25 years in Jail"

"Local cult preacher Father Hotep or 'Big Daddy Hotep' as he was called by his followers aka Duke Preston, of the Temple of Everlasting Faith, in Patchogue, L.I., was arrested today on charges of tax evasion and child molestation. Teenage girls as young as fourteen years old had been forced to stay and live in the temple's residences while being subjected to various forms of mind control, drug abuse and group sex for over ten years.

Followers were forced to give up their money and work long hours selling merchandise they had produced in factories run by Father Hotep.

When asked why he, supposedly a man of God, would do this to his followers Father Hotep said frankly: 'Those girls opened their legs to me...I didn't force them to do anything against their will.

You know young girls these days, they're nasty, and they don't know what's good for them. They only know what makes them feel good, and, I made them feel good!'

Father Hotep, was released on a $250,000 bond and is living somewhere on Long Island awaiting trial."

The rumors were definitely true. I was so relieved that the truth had finally been revealed because, like my mother had always said: **"There ain't nothing the devil does in the dark that doesn't one day come to the light."** My Mommy was always right. Another one of her famous sayings was: **"If I tell you it's Christmas, then you'd better hang up your stocking and call me Santa."** It was Christmas for me. This meant that I wouldn't have to pay Duke back. I guess Duke's luck had finally run out. I felt bad for him, but I also couldn't help but wonder how such an intelligent and handsome man could lose his way and sink into such a cesspool of a life.

I heard the mailman pull up to my house and went outside to meet him.

"Hey…Willie…what's good today?"

"Oh hey, Miss C.J.…nice to see you again. You're looking real good these days! Got a letter for you from New York. Sorry to hear that you were in the hospital."

"I'm feeling much better now, thank you. Lost a little weight, too…couldn't you tell?"

"I sure could…So, tell your husband to watch out! I just might try to steal you away from him!"

"Oh, Willie…you're such a flatterer."

Willie had been our mailman ever since we moved to Atlanta. He knew practically everything about me and was a good friend, besides. He handed me the mail and took off down the block in his truck. I briefly looked at the envelopes and saw one from the hospital in New York. Thinking that it was the bill, and wanting to see how much it was, I opened the envelope right there on the sidewalk outside my front door. When I saw what was in the letter I almost fainted.

Dr. Kirkpatrick had made an appointment for me to see one of his colleagues at the local University Hospital in Athens, Georgia to discuss the status of my HIV tests. He urged me to keep this appointment and to make sure I took all of the proper precautions to prevent the further spread of the virus. HIV tests? I didn't even know they had taken an HIV test in New York. And, exactly what was my status?

The letter did not divulge that information. The appointment was for that Thursday at 1:00 PM, but I couldn't wait that long. I got on the phone and called Dr. Kirkpatrick's office immediately. I got his colleague Dr. Maney.

"Dr. Maney...what does it mean in this letter from your office about the status of my HIV tests. Did you all do an HIV test without my knowledge?"

"Why, Yes, Mrs. Greene...those tests are standard procedure in all emergency rooms these days to protect the providers from handling dangerous bodily fluids. We need to know the status of our patients if they are unable to speak for themselves so that we can take the proper precautions. Like I said before, it's standard procedure."

"I understand standard procedures, but is it standard procedure to not tell your patients the results of their tests right away?"

"Mrs. Greene, please calm down. You were in no condition to handle this type of news."

"What news doctor...what are you trying to say? Spit it out, man!"

"You tested positive...Mrs. Greene." I held the phone in my hand without speaking for what seemed to be an eternity." Hello...Mrs. Greene, are you still there? Hello...hello...?"

I dropped the phone and sat on the steps; staring into space for about a minute. Finally, I answered the doctor who was still holding on the phone. My voice shook uncontrollably.

"I see,...Dr. Maney...Um...Dr. Maney, I have to go now. I will talk to you and Dr. Kirkpatrick later, O.K.?"

"I understand, Mrs. Greene. Please be well. Goodbye."

All I could think about was what I was going to tell my family?

Should I keep it a secret and act like nothing had happened or should I come clean with the news? How could I tell my children that their mother was infected with a deadly disease and that she could die soon? How could I tell my husband that I may have infected him and that we were possibly not going to be together until we were old and gray? My husband...my loving and wonderful husband...I had to speak to him, immediately and find out what was going on.

I dialed his cell phone and he picked up immediately.

"Sly...I...I...need to...talk to you...Baby!" I could barely breathe or speak as the tears came rolling down my face.

"C.J....what happened?" he asked, excitedly.

"I got a letter from the hospital....and..." I choked.

"I know...baby, I know."

"What do you mean, you know?"

"They told me in New York. Jesus, C.J. --- I didn't want it to be like this. I was hoping I could come home sooner and spend some time with you, before you found out."

"You knew? You knew and you didn't tell me? You knew and you didn't tell me? I never want to speak to you ever again in life!"

I hung up the phone and when he called back I just let it ring. I went straight to my liquor cabinet and searched for the half empty bottle of Brandy that I had left over for special occasions. **'This is a special occasion'**, I thought, opened the bottle, poured a big glass of the brown liquid and downed it in two or three gulps. I finished the rest of the bottle and soon I had passed out on my bed. I didn't even hear my son come home from school. He thought I was taking a nap and just went to his room to do his homework.

Chapter 14

Factuality

When you have seen as much of life as I have, you will
not underestimate the power of obsessive love.

J. K. Rowling Harry Potter and the Half-Blood Prince, 2005

I immediately sunk into a depression that you
could not imagine. Marcella came down from New York
to help me take care of Milo, who kept asking me what
was wrong with me. All I could tell him was that his
Mommy was sick and that I couldn't take care of him.
Sylvester immediately flew home from California to be
by my side, but I was oblivious to his presence.

I stayed angry and I couldn't talk to anyone for
over three days. I couldn't eat and I could barely pull
myself out of bed to go to the bathroom. There was only
so much I could feel at that time. I was numb to the
bone. Every day that I was alive was a blessing, but I

couldn't see it that way. I stayed in bed for over a week and I missed the first doctor's appointment.

The girls on the job took over my duties like champions. I had hired talented and responsible women and they stepped up to the plate to take care of the business; knowing full well that I was in no shape to do anything but try to cope with living each day. Everyone was careful to not say or do anything that would upset me, and they just allowed me to exist in that state.

Until one day, something hit me--- and I decided that I was going to do whatever it took to beat the disease. I was not going to allow it to beat me! I got up and started looking for information about HIV and AIDS on the Internet.

The money in the bank was a little comfort, but I kept thinking **what good was money if I wasn't going to be alive to spend it?** I had to do everything in my power to overcome this cruel blow that Fate had dealt to me. The first thing I needed to do was find out how I got the virus.

I started doing the calculations in my head. Sylvester and I had been married a little over eight months. We both had gotten complete STD screenings before we got married as required by the state. I usually got tested every year like clockwork.

So, either one of us had become infected *just prior* to getting tested last year, or Sylvester wasn't telling me the whole truth about his extramarital affairs. I found out that there is about a six week "incubation" period before you body shows indications of being infected.

He was due to go back to California on the weekend, so I had to find out what was really going on right away. That Friday, I awoke early, got up, took my shower and went into the kitchen to make myself a cup of coffee, as usual. My son came into the kitchen and was extremely happy to see me.

"Hey, Mommy!...You're up! Are you feeling better now?"

"I'm feeling so much better, Pumpkin. You just go on to school, and I will be right here waiting for you when you get home, alright?" I could not imagine not being around to see him go to college. Marcella came into the room behind him.

"I'm glad to see you up and around, Mommy. That means you're getting stronger."

"I am *much stronger* now, Marcy. I did a lot of soul searching and praying in that bed upstairs and I've come to the conclusion that I have w-a-ay too much to live for to let this thing get me down. They have a lot of new treatments these days and I can live a rich full life. I don't have to be an invalid if I don't' want to."

"Now that's the spirit...because I am losing *a hell of a lot of money*, and I gotta get back to my shop or else I'll be out of business in a New York minute."

"Yes, baby…you go on back to New York to take care of Darice. Don't worry about that money. I will take care of you. Momma is gonna be just fine!"

I gave her a big hug and saw Sly standing in the doorway behind her with his suitcase next to him.

"Were you just going to leave without saying goodbye, again?"

"No, Sugar…That's why I came down to find you."

"Good…because you know we need to talk…"

Marcella cut in. "I'll just take Milo to school and I'll talk to you later, Mom, O.K.? Come on short stuff…let's go."

"That's fine, Marcy. I'll see you guys later. Sly--- have a seat, Darlin'…We need to talk right now."

"But, my plane leaves in two hours…" he was trying to avoid the inevitable.

"Book…a later flight," I said slowly "…this is more important."

He sat down at the counter and I fixed him a cup of coffee, while we talked.

"Sylvester, my dearest…I married you because, I thought that I loved you and I thought that you loved me, too."

"I do love you, C.J.….you know that."

"Well then…let's take a little trip down memory lane and see what sites we run into along the way, OK?. Now--- we both had STD screenings before we got married, right?"

'Um, hum…" He looked at the floor and fiddled nervously with his coffee.

"And, both of our tests came up negative, right?"

'Um, hum…"

"Therefore, either the tests were wrong...or one of us hasn't been telling the *whole truth*! Am I correct?"

"You are correct as usual, C.J." He was looking *really* guilty at that point.

"Now before you go traipsing off to California to take care of business,--- is there anything you want to tell me?"

"C.J....I want to tell you that I can fix this...but I can't! I want to tell you that sometimes people do things that they wish they hadn't done, but it's too late to fix things and they have to just do the best that they can to move on."

"Sylvester Greene...we are not kids anymore. I am a grown woman and you are a grown man. I know that we are both human, and we're not perfect, either. Stop beating around the bush and tell me what it is you are trying to say. Spit it out, Man!"

"You were in Africa, Baby…you were gone for like two whole weeks and…" he began. He was talking so fast the words seem to come out of his mouth in one long sentence.

"And…?"

"And, Steve came over and asked me to go to the club with him to get me out of the house for a little while and I swear…I didn't plan for it to happen… C.J."

"You didn't plan for what to happen, Sly? You'd better tell me what you did!!"

He started to sob softly as he spoke.

"After we left the club he took me to his friend's house and his friend had another friend there, and we were watching videos, and…Oh, God…C.J.…I told you, I ain't no punk,… I ain't no punk, C.J.… you weren't here… and I needed you to be here to hold me, C.J.…I needed you so bad…I needed you, and, and…"

"And you had sex with that girl, didn't you?" He nodded his head.

"That damned Steve! I knew he was no good for you! Did you at least use a condom?"

He nodded his head. "It broke..."

"Oh my sweet, Jesus..." I said, and got up to pace the floor. "And, you never told me?"

"I didn't tell you because I was scared to death, Baby. I got a problem...I...I thought that getting married would cure me. "

"Yeah...you got a real big problem now, don't you?"

I was amazingly calm for someone who had just been told that she had contracted a deadly disease from some stinking whore who didn't have the decency to leave a married man alone. But, I had a few secrets of my own under my belt so I could only get but so angry.

"Sly...we have to go to the doctor and make sure the tests have been confirmed. I'm not perfect either...and since we are playing 'Truth, or

Consequences, Promise or Repeat' ... I have a little confession of my own to make."

Sly raised his head and looked at me curiously while I paced the floor nervously.

"Look...I wasn't such an angel when I went to Africa, either. I went out to dinner with my client, the King... I got a little tipsy and when he took me back to my hotel room, ...and...and... things kind of got out of hand. We didn't go all the way...I mean, ...I stopped him before we actually got it on, ... but we were going at it for about a good five or ten minutes. I was horny and kind of missing you, too. So, I guess I kinda understand what you were going through. But, we both have a serious problem now, Sly. What are we going to do about this?"

"You had sex with the King?" he asked, with a straight face.

"You know they believe in polygamy over there. He was going to make a big investment in the company. At least I was going to get some money out of the deal!"

"C.J....that's called Prostitution, --- that's not an investment."

"You call it whatever you want. At least we used a condom...and, and... it didn't break!"

"So, I guess we're even now, huh?" Sly asked.

"I guess so...so what are we going to do about this problem, now?"

"I guess I'll tell Steve to take care of his own business and I'll stay here and take care of my wife," he said.

"No...first you come on go with me to get the instant HIV test, then you go on to California and do whatever it is you gotta do and I'll stay here and do whatever it is I gotta do. You stay out of Steve's apartment, don't watch any more of those damned videos, and you call me every day, twice a day...three times a day...as many times a day that you feel you need to call me...And, in a couple of months you'll come back home, we'll be together for the holidays and we'll have a wonderfully good time together as man and wife! Now come here and give me some sugar."

"C.J....You are an amazing woman...I guess that's why I married you!"

"No...you married me 'cause I'm so good to you."

"You got that right," he agreed an gave me a big kiss.

He went off to California and I got busy back in my design shop. Our life seemed to settle down a bit right before the big storm hit. We were about to be tested beyond belief.

Chapter 15

Quality

In battling evil, excess is good; for he who is moderate in
announcing the truth is presenting half-truth.

He conceals the other half out of fear of the people's
wrath.

Kahlil Gibran (1883 - 1931), *'Narcotics and Dissecting*
Knives, Thoughts and Meditations

In the ensuing months, I had to make several
extremely important decisions; not only about how I was
going to deal with living with the HIV virus, but how I
was going to deal with living in a world full of people who
either took these matters so nonchalantly, and then
treated people with HIV like proverbial pariahs. Life is
short and life is precious and we should never take life
for granted because like my cousin Josephine said at my
mother's funeral: **"You never know when it is going
to be your turn next."** We must live our lives as if

each day were our last. We must also be mindful of the things that we do today, –- for tomorrow is not promised to any of us. Wrong decisions, angry words, deceptions, grudges, careless actions...all these things diminish the quality of our lives and leave us no room for health, love and happiness to grow.

I am quite sure that the young girls (or whomever he said was a girl) who threw themselves at my husband, and those who succumbed to the false teachings of Duke Preston, never stopped to consider what effect their actions would have on their futures. That is supposed to be the difference between the young and the old. Old people have developed something called "foresight" from being around for so long. Young people sometimes can't see past their noses in the dark.

If you are smart, you can understand that five or ten minutes of pleasure can lead to *a lifetime* of pain and misery that is not worth it in the long run.

If you are dumb or weak you will allow yourself to be over-taken by your physical feelings or your emotions and you'll do something that you will regret forever!

I don't even know whether or not my husband ever told the person that he was with that he was married. Most of the time men don't say anything because they know that if they did, the girls would not have sex with them. On the other hand, there are those people who don't care who they have sex with, because they are just out to get laid, like the girl who was after my daughter's boyfriend.

Young people no longer care about what type of "reputation" they develop. On the contrary, the nastier they are the more popular they become. Women lose their "virtue" at a seemingly younger and younger age these days, and I doubt that the young men they socialize with truly respect them, at all.

Men will sleep with those naïve young women, then turn around and call them "skank whores" behind their backs. Then marry the ones who don't go to bed with them right away, or they'll marry the ones who go to church all the time and have kept their virginity for marriage. Men have an entirely different take on sex than women do.

Men basically can have sex *for a physical release only!* It is a primal instinct to them. They can have sex with a woman, (a dog, a man, a sheep, a prostitute, a slut, whatever) get up, wash off, and go back home to their wives and their families without remorse. **It is truly a big deal for a man to say that he loves you,** because he must use his mind (his big head, so to speak) to *think about the woman* for whom he has special feelings. When a woman has sex with a man it is an entirely different story.

Women are usually looking for true love ---Usually! A woman who has sex with a man she barely knows is usually looking for something other than the pure physical release. She is either looking for the attention, (because she has low self-esteem, and needs to be reassured that she is beautiful or worthy of a man's attention), emotional comfort (because she thinks that having sex is equivalent to making love…same actions, but different results), or some type of reward (money, fame, or conquest, etc. ("Nah, nah…I took your man, so what?")

And, I can understand the pressures that these women are under to have sex because that is all they see in the media. They don't see women being praised for being virtuous. They only see the attention that men give them for being "nasty girls."

However, they also don't see what happens to those women after they have thrown themselves away to men who couldn't care less about them in the long run. Twenty or thirty years down the road, they end up lonely and alone because men still don't truly respect women who are "easy".

At the end of the day, men are still hunters who truly appreciate a woman who can give him "a run for his money", and are a "challenge". They may *have sex* with the easy girls, but they *marry and keep* the ones who are not.

It is usually very hard for a woman to have sex without being emotional; almost as difficult it is for a man to have emotions without wanting to have sex. Centuries of men being forced to have sex outside of marriage (through war, business, or egotistical conquests) have allowed them to develop insensitivity to their own emotions.

Unfortunately, women are still the one's to have babies, still are very emotional beings, and **unprotected sex still leads to unwanted pregnancies.** And, the fact that these women are having sex is not truly the issue.

The issue is that they are having **UNPROTECTED SEX!**

Without condoms and without reliable birth control; they are setting themselves up for all kinds of venereal diseases and death, and then bringing young children into the mix, thus perpetuating the whole nasty cycle over and over again. Thus, we are back to the point I was trying to make in the beginning:

Women must not allow men to take advantage of their bodies without taking responsibility for the results of their actions.

There is an old Chinese saying: **"No need for rape...Woman run faster with dress up, than man do with pants down."** Thus, confirming the fact that women totally control the sexual nature and outcome of their lives and the morality of society at large. Women must be the ones to save the race from total destruction from sexually transmitted diseases.

I decided to stay with my husband because I realized that if I left him:

1. I would have a very hard time finding another man who would not only want to be with an older woman, but

who also wanted to be with an older woman who had the AIDS virus.

2. If we got a divorce I would have to give him half of my money, liquidate my assets and move out of my home. As long as we stayed together, I could put off telling him about the Lotto money and safely use it to finance my business.

3. I, too, was guilty of infidelity, and he could have divorced me just as easily. (ie. two wrongs don't make a right). If he wanted to stay, I wasn't going to chase him away.

4. The stress of another divorce trial probably would have literally killed me. I needed to get healthy and not have a lot of anger and resentment building up inside of me.

5. My children would have been traumatized again by seeing their mother suffering and I would probably would have died of a heart attack or a stroke at an early age.

I had a lot of fences to mend and very little time in which to do it. The first fence I needed to mend was the one between me and my daughter, Joanna. She had gone back to school, and I hadn't the slightest idea how what was going on in *my* life was affecting *her*. She was about to go through her mid-term exams and I was quite sure she was having an extremely hard time concentrating on her studies.

It had to have been almost a month since she had returned to Philadelphia and I realized that I hadn't heard from her. I had been so caught up in my own pain and suffering, I realized that we hadn't even had a decent conversation since the funeral. I called her cell phone and left several message for her. After about ten messages she finally called me back but was cold as ice.

"Mommy...it's Joanna. How are you? What do you want?"

"How am I? How are you doing, Darlin'? And I want to apologize to you."

"I'm doing alright, Mommy. But, Shawn and I broke up. "

"Why did y'all break up?"

"Just like you said, Mommy...he was just taking advantage of me. He moved into my room and all he did was expect me to cook, have sex, *and* clean up after him. He didn't even want to give me any money and I had to pay for the room and all the food. I couldn't get any of my studying done and finally I told him that he was going to have to leave."

"That's my girl..." She was beginning to warm up to me.

"And, besides that, the girl his roommate and his roommate's girlfriend were fighting over was trying to get with Shawn, too. She was just a piece of nasty trash who was hanging out over there trying to get laid every night. And, I caught Shawn kissing her, too!"

"Well...I'm glad you made the right decision, Hon. What did I do to deserve such a wonderful child?"

"Mom...I'm sorry I cursed at you and got mad at you. You haven't been such a bad parent, after all. You did your best. I know that Daddy was a big dog back in the day...He put you through a lot.

You were really a good singer, too, and he just couldn't appreciate someone being more talented than he was. I remember some of them girls he used to bring to the house when you were out on the road. He used to try to make me call them 'Auntie'...and some of them... ugh...were really ugly, too! It was disgusting!"

"Oh no, he didn't..." I was in shock. "Why didn't you ever tell me this?"

"I really didn't remember until now...it was a long time ago." She paused. "So, what are you going to do about the virus, Mommy?"

"I'm seeing a doctor and I'm taking my pills. I'm thinking about getting a naturopath."

"What's a naturopath?" She asked.

"You know a *wholistic doctor;* one who uses herbs and vitamins and juices and stuff and who can really take care of my mind, body and spirit."

"Don't worry, Mommy...we'll get through this together. So do you know how you got it? Was it Sly?"

"Joanna---now that's really none of your business. Sylvester and I have a lot of stuff to work out in our lives together. It's not that simple. I would just hope that you have gotten tested and that you know your own status, and then, once you know... you'll do everything in *your power* to maintain your status which hopefully will be negative for the rest of your life."

"Don't worry...my Momma didn't raise no fool! I already got tested and I'm just fine."

"Make me proud, Baby...Good luck on your midterms. We'll see you on Thanksgiving, alright?"

"Alright, Mommy...I love you."

"I love you too, baby...see you soon. Bye."

There are a lot of things in this world that truly disturb me. One of these things is the way that young people float in and out of relationships, and have sex with different people the way that they change their outfits. There is no more sincerity or fidelity. They lie, cheat and play shameless mind games with each other's emotions like they are on some kind of soap opera, sit com, or game show on television.

I believe that what is going on is a direct result of the so-called Sexual Revolution of the eighties and nineties and the fact that people have casual sex like they are riding a roller coaster in an amusement park. True morality is dead, there is no more love or affection for one another, and the way that people act is just plain disgusting.

I don't know if it is worse these days or if it was worse back in the Seventies when the Sexual Revolution began. At least back in those days if your "one night stand" chose to stick around for a few months, or if you had sex with a guy for more than a month, you were in a relationship and usually ended up married.

Nowadays, people have multiple sex partners, have no idea who the fathers of their children are, suffer from horrendous sexually transmitted diseases like Chlamydia, herpes, genital warts, and even Syphilis is making a strong comeback.

You see them on talk shows and court TV acting like total idiots airing their shameful dirty laundry like insidious badges of dishonor. It is also the results of children raising children and the destruction of the family from divorce and casual dating.

What can a twenty-five year old teach a twelve year old, if she had the baby when she was just thirteen years old herself, and she is now sharing her bed every night with one or several of her boyfriends? What was going on in her life that made her choose having sex and making a baby as opposed to getting an education, going to college, and finding a decent job or a decent husband?

What values was her mother, (that is, if her mother was around at all) teaching her at that tender young age? Or, was her mother too busy, too occupied, too stressed out, too drugged up, too overwhelmed, or too uneducated to do a proper job of raising a child into adulthood, herself? How do you learn how to be a good parent when you are only thirteen years old?

The parenting skills of adults in our society are totally appalling. They either allow their children to do whatever they want to, or they are so strict that the children either develop complexes, obsessive compulsive disorders, or they totally break free the first chance they get and become absolutely uncontrollable, dysfunctional adults.

There are parenting magazines, books, pamphlets, classes, and seminars, yet the children are still out of control and disrespectful of authority because their parents are too lazy, ignorant or unconcerned to learn how to parent properly. Then the parents try to buy their children's love with expensive toys, clothing and other indulgences thinking that money can make their children behave and grow up to be productive members of society.

There are no more defined boundaries for what is appropriate for children to see or hear or wear and the results are the "inmates running the asylum" mentality of families in our society. And, then we wonder why crime, decadence and disease are so commonplace.

How did my friend, Duke, take a positive message and turn it into one of the most heinous forms of manipulation one could ever practice? How can teachers, scout leaders, preachers, priests and nuns, and some other adults take advantage of children by molesting them, putting them into pornographic, sexually explicit videos or other forms of sexual media?

It's because our children are looking for attention, love and affection. Where they would normally get those things from their parents, it seems that parents are too busy these days making money or "doing their own thing" to worry or to care about what is going on with their children

Sexual predators know this and prey on children who have no strong foundations in their lives..

So, where are the adults in the society to say:

"You know what? We've had enough of this!"

How many more of our children must die a horrible death from suicide, child abuse, drug overdoses, or venereal diseases, because no adult was brave enough to stand up and say:

"Save our children, NOW!"

Well, I've had enough! I would never allow my children to be subjected to the horrors of child pornography, early drug abuse or abandonment of my parental duties. I care about them too much to destroy their futures like that.

It is abandonment when a parent allows a stranger to have more of an influence over their child than they do. It is abandonment when a parent doesn't have the foresight to know that their child is in trouble and headed for a brick wall in life. And, it is abandonment when a parent does not take lessons or acquire the information necessary to lead their children in the right direction in life.

It is child abuse when a parent doesn't realize how what they are doing affects their children's lives.

There should be laws against some of the things that parents do (or don't do) to their children these days, but unfortunately there aren't and it isn't until the child commits a crime, runs away from home, or is found dead somewhere that something is said about the abusive bad parenting that children are subjected to in their homes. Unfortunately, most bad parenting skills don't cause the physical scars that are punishable by the law and the mental scars are merely passed on to the next generation of bad parents.

AIDS is the plague that God has sent to us to make us take heed and do something to save our children before it is too late. There was a reason why sex was kept away from children back in the day. Our children are suffering and dying today, because we have allowed them to do as they please without restraint.

There was a reason why sex was supposed to be practiced within the confines of marriage, and marriage alone, by mature committed adults.

It's because extramarital sexual activities lead to corruption, disease and devastation. And, minors cannot handle the emotional consequences of having sex

During a recent blood drive, they had to discard over 40% of the blood collected because it had been found to be contaminated with the HIV. That means that in another 10 or 15 years a major portion of our young people will never reach adulthood. And, if they do, they will be invalids living a miserable life with full blown AIDS.

They will be a drain on society and our health care system will be crippled, if something is not done NOW!

This story does not have a happy ending. I wish I could tell you that it did. I have to tell you what happened to all of the money...

Chapter 16

The Reality

Wise men profit more from fools than fools from wise men; for the wise men shun the mistakes of fools, but fools do not imitate the successes of the wise.

Cato the Elder (234 BC - 149 BC), *from Plutarch, Lives*

Thanksgiving came, Sylvester came home from California, Joanna came home from school, and Marcella drove down to Atlanta to have dinner with the family. It had been a while since we had learned the news of my having the HIV virus and the others were becoming curious about how Sylvester and I were coping with the change in our health status. The conversation at the dinner table was strained and forced.

"So...Mommy...um...how are you and Sylvester feeling these days?" Marcella asked.

"We're feeling just fine, thank you for asking. We're taking our meds, eating healthy and we're dealing with it."

"Marcella, your mother and I have gone through a lot together and I think this whole situation has made our love for one another stronger. Wouldn't you agree, C.J.?" Sylvester remarked.

"Oh most definitely…We still have few issues to work on but, generally we're coping," I agreed.

"So, Mom…have you told Sylvester about…you know,…*the ticket?*" Marcella asked; winking her eye at me.

"What ticket?" asked Sly.

"Oh…she's talking about the ticket I just bought to go to India," I said smiling broadly, as I kicked Marcella under the table. "My client wants us to do their house in an Eastern theme and I have to go to Calcutta to get some stuff. I won't be away long…just three or four days a the most."

"Do you think you're strong enough to fly overseas? Don't they make you take special shots, and stuff? Why do you have to go right now?" he asked.

"Oh, my doctor is going to give me a special clearance. I'll be fine! And, it's just for a few days, so I'll be back before you even know I am gone."

Now I either had to really go to India or come up with some excuse as to why I *wasn't* going. (You see how when you lie, you have to just keep adding to the lies?) I had to explain to Marcella that the money was being held in my corporate account until I could decide how I was going to spend it. In the meanwhile, I had to resist the urge to go shopping, to buy a new car, go to Europe on an expensive vacation or do any of those kinds of things, because *$250,000 really doesn't go very far.* And, if I wasn't careful I could end up dead broke in a nursing home. The knowledge that my money could help repair my marriage and possibly buy us some more time on this earth together was more than I could ever hope for. I had planned to tell my husband, *eventually.*

Unfortunately, again, as Fate would have it God had a different plan for my life.

I decided that I would find out about all of the wholistic doctors in India who could give us information and cures for HIV. I probably could have found one here in the United States, but I thought that a trip overseas would give me a sort of vacation, and time to recharge my batteries. I planned to go after the holidays during the slow season, and I would tell Sly about the money when I got back.

I was sitting at my desk in my design studio one day right before the holidays. The girls had gone out to lunch and I was flipping through some travel brochures and some gift catalogs; trying to decide what I was going to buy the kids for Christmas. Just then, I heard the wind chimes at the front door of the shop telling me that I had a visitor.

286

"I'll be right there," I yelled out.

"Don't get up on my account," said a familiar voice. It was Duke in a dirty, scummy looking sweat suit with about three days worth of beard on his face.

"Oh my God..." I whispered. "Duke, how did you find me?"

He looked around the office carefully.

"Nice place you got here. You're doing very well for yourself if I must say so, *Mrs. Greene*. It took me a while to find you but I did finally...Greene's Art Deco and Design... right there in the Yellow Pages...You couldn't help using your married name, now could you? Being married always meant so much to you, didn't it?"

"Duke...Why did you come here?"

"Like I told your husband...we have some unfinished business to take care of," he said, with his teeth clenched tightly.

"Look, if you're talking about the hospital bill, I can write you a check right now," I said, and pulled out my company's checkbook from inside my desk drawer.

"What the hell am I going to do with your funky little check, Miss C.J.? They froze my bank accounts and confiscated my assets, Bitch! I don't want your freaking check! No,--- *we are* going to take a little trip to the bank and get some cold, hard cash, Baby. Come on, let's go!"

He pulled out a gun from his jacket pocket and pointed it straight at my head. I nearly fainted dead on the spot.

'Oh, my God…Duke, please don't do this!" I pleaded with him.

"COME ON!!" he yelled and grabbed me by the arm. "We're going for a little ride. Get your bag!"

Outside, a car was waiting with a young lady in the driver's seat. He opened the back door and threw me inside. I almost hit my head on the roof of the car.

"Let's go, Leticia. Tell her where to go, C.J."

"Go down to the end of the block and make a right."

We headed for the center of town towards my bank. Then, I told him:

"Duke, you'll never get away with this, you know. They will find you."

"SHUT UP!" he yelled, and backhanded me across the mouth. *"I am not* going back to jail! --- Been there done that, remember? I will die before I let them put me back in that hell hole. You are going to take out $10,000 cash and me, Leticia here, and you are going to go to Mexico for a little vacation. Ain't that right, Leticia?"

"That's right, Big Daddy..." she answered.

"Leticia...this is not a movie! This is real life, girl, you can go to jail for this!"

"Didn't I tell you to shut up?" Duke hit me again so hard that my head hit the window. The pain shot down my neck. "Now tell her where to go..."

"Make a left at the intersection."

We finally reached the bank. Duke made me get out and go inside while Leticia waited in the car. Suddenly, I realized that I had my cell phone in my pocket and I pushed the #5 button for my quick dial programmed number to 911. Then, I then prayed that the police would hear everything that was going on, and I made sure to talk loud enough to let them know that I was in trouble.

"Duke...Please...Don't do this... You are going to just make things worse!"

He held me close to him with one hand and aimed the gun hidden in his pocket at my ribs. We walked into the bank and headed for the customer service area to make the withdrawal.

"Good afternoon, Mrs. Greene…so nice to see you! What can we do for you this afternoon?"

The nice customer service representative waived us over to sit down at her desk. I tried to act cool and nonchalant and hide my swollen cheek behind my hand. My hands were shaking violently as I tried to find a pen in my purse.

"Um…I need to make a withdrawal. A rather large withdrawal that is," I began, trying to look as nonchalant as possible.

"Alright then, let me just get a slip here…" She reached into her desk and pulled out a checking withdrawal slip.

I pretended to fill it out but instead I wrote very quickly: "**HELP ME!**" Then I handed the slip back to her. Duke jumped up quickly. He pulled the gun out of his waistband.

"You double crossing bitch…I oughta blow your ass away right now!"
He fired a shot into the air.

"EVERYBODY HIT THE FLOOR RIGHT NOW!!" he yelled, grabbed me by the arm, and pulled me to the middle of the floor.

"DON'T NOBODY MOVE OR I WILL BLOW HER HEAD OFF RIGHT NOW! GET ME ALL THE MONEY FROM THE DRAWERS...NOW!"

The tellers started emptying their tills into bags, but within seconds we heard a police siren off in the distance outside. Duke grabbed a bag from the first and second tellers while dragging me along next to him. I struggled to get away, and he couldn't handle me, the gun and the money bags, so when we got near the door he let me go, and turned to run. He stopped short, turned back, and shot me near my right shoulder. I fell to the floor in agony.

"That's for being such a bitch!" he said as he ran out to the car where Leticia was waiting. I could hear the tires screeching and gunshots being fired as the people in the bank ran over to me.

"Someone call 911..." I heard the customer service woman who had just waited on me say right before I passed out.

I told you that this story did not have a happy ending.

Duke and Leticia were killed by the cops when they tried to escape in a high speed chase through Atlanta. They killed an old woman who was crossing the street near the bank and destroyed several parked cars in the wake of the chase. They ended up wrapped around a pole on the highway.

All of the young people who lived in the big house on the hill in Patchogue were forced to move out and find other homes when Duke's church was closed up. They found out that Duke had had over twenty young children by different girls from the church who were then left without a father and no means of support. Leticia's six month old baby was left to be a ward of the State in Foster Care.

I spent six weeks in the hospital recuperating. My body was not strong enough to fight the gunshot wound, and my HIV got worse. Since I was not home to take care of my family, and could not afford full time childcare, the burden of my son's care fell on my ex-husband. My son had to be uprooted to go live with his father in California for the holidays which then turned into a permanent situation. I lost the $10,000 in tuition money for his private school and he lost his placement for the next semester. My hospital and nursing home care bill came to just over $150,000.

My daughter Joanna flunked out of her first semester of school from all of the stress and distractions. She eventually went back, but she was so far behind that they had to put her on academic probation for the rest of the year. She also went back to her boyfriend, for comfort, and she got pregnant the next year. She didn't have the baby, but the whole ordeal cost me over $45,000 for the lost semesters of work and the hospital care for her abortion.

They got into a big fight one night over money and where they were going to live. Shawn beat her up and cut her face, and he is now spending five years in jail for the assault. She lost a pending modeling contract and her dreams of going to Paris vanished overnight.

Since he had acquired a criminal record, Shawn got kicked out of school permanently. His roommate and his roommate's girlfriend had to move into a homeless shelter when they couldn't find another place to live. Her four year old daughter came to visit her one weekend and was raped by a teenage boy who lived in the shelter, who had some serious mental problems. The little girl is now in therapy for acting out in sexual play with the other little boys who lived in her neighborhood. She is now damaged for life and will never be the same.

Joanna decided to drop out of school for the next year, and I haven't heard from her in months. Marcella tells me that she calls her periodically and she thinks that she is living with a pimp somewhere in Atlanta. She is a smart girl and I just pray that she doesn't let my illness affect her for very long. I pray that she will get the therapy she needs to learn how to cope with the anger that she feels about my situation.

My husband, Sly, had *another* affair with someone he'd met in California, whom he had turned to for comfort, because I was not there to take care of him. At least that's what he told me... But, the girl turned out to be a man! It was Steve, his best friend. He wrote me a letter one day to tell me about it.

Dearest C. J., my love...

I am so sorry I had to put you through this. When I met you I truly thought that we were going to be together forever until we died. I never thought that it would be like this. I always loved you, you know that. But, I also loved someone else before you came into my life. Steve wasn't just my business partner he was my lover, too. It all started a long time ago and I never had the nerve to tell you, about us. He was always there for me when you weren't. He knew that I couldn't tell anyone about us so he agreed to keep the secret from you, too.

I had a lot of problems, C.J. You would never have understood all that I have been through over the years. I know you tried your best, but sometimes your best just isn't good enough. My homo-sexuality or bisexuality or whatever you want to call it--- was a demon to me. I didn't know how to deal with it like other people do. I fought that demon my whole life, but I guess he won.

I tried to be the man that you needed me to be, but I couldn't even be the man that I needed me to be for myself. I am truly sorry for everything, but I just couldn't take the pain or the guilt anymore.

Always your man, Sly

When Steve had found out about his HIV status, he sued him for over $100,000 for deception, pain and suffering. He had to leave California, and the limo business failed completely. He came back to Atlanta a broken man, decided that he couldn't live with the guilt of possibly having given me the HIV virus and having lost all of his money. In his depression he committed suicide from an overdose of painkillers and sleeping pills!

His letter also confessed to me that his bad dreams were cause by the fact that he had killed a man for raping him when he was in his teens, and had spent ten years in a juvenile detention center where he was molested and beat up daily by one of the other inmates who was much larger and older than he was. But he had turned to one of the other inmates for comfort and protection and they had a homosexual relationship for over five years.

He had never told me about this because he was ashamed about his past and thought that I wouldn't marry him if I knew what he had been through. He suffered miserably with the guilt of having caused my illness, but I didn't have the heart and never got the chance to tell him that I had lied about using a condom when I had sex with the King in Africa. We didn't use a condom that night at all. I lied because I was scared, and I had just read in the papers about the area of Africa where I visited has a 50% incidence of HIV infections among the population there.

Although, my business was starting to do well at the time, I had lost all my clients because I was not there to run it anymore. I had to lay off all my employees and through Unemployment Insurance I had to pay them over $10,000 each until they found new jobs. I eventually had to sell the business and liquidate my assets just to keep afloat. When I was finally discharged from the nursing home, I had a little over $50,000 left in the bank.

With the lack of insurance monies after my husband's death, which I couldn't claim was accidental because of the suicide note he left, I had to pay over $10,000 in cash for his funeral and final expenses. I lost the use of my right arm and could no longer do my artwork or cut fabric. I was literally back to square one in my Life.

I managed to get a little bit better, but I am not totally well, not by a long shot. I eventually sold my big house in Atlanta and moved to a little bungalow in Baltimore with my cousin. I couldn't work for a while, and I struggled with the AIDS virus for another year, until one day my doctor told me that my "T " cell count had improved slightly and it appeared that the HIV was in remission. I now live off of a small Social Security Disability check, but it is nothing like the thousands of dollars I used to make in a month. Without a husband or other emotional support, I feel totally lost.

I am still so lonely and miserable, that it's practically unbearable. I drink myself to sleep almost every night, although taking alcohol is against my doctor's orders. I don't date because I am afraid of what will happen if a man finds out that I have the virus. My cousin is also HIV positive, and we give each other moral support to keep living day by day, but he is much sicker than I am and the doctor says that he may die very soon. I don't know what I am going to do without him.

My son is afraid to touch me when he comes to visit, for fear that he will get sick, too. He thinks that I abandoned him, and that I didn't want him around me anymore and that is the reason why I sent him to California to live with his Dad. He is full of anger and confusion and doesn't really understand my illness, but he thinks like most other people that I am contagious and won't touch anything that I have touched. The only one who will give me hugs is my daughter Marcella, who is still my rock despite all the things I have put her through in her life.

Today I am an AIDS/HIV counselor in my local rehab center in Baltimore where I live with one of my cousins who also has AIDS.. A life of riches and fame is the furthest thing from my mind. The stress in my life is so enormous that I cry all the time. My life will never be the same again, because I lost my home, my husband, my business, my money, and I almost lost my children, again.

I still haven't heard from Joanna, but I hear from Marcella that, at least she is alive. I, on the other hand, may die in another year and I may live for another twenty. We don't know for sure. I live each day as it comes and I say a prayer for each day that I am still alive.

But, I need you to understand that it was all because---- although we were adults, we had made all the wrong decisions! All the pain and misery we suffered could have easily been avoided if we only knew better!

I never dreamed that a mistake in *my life* could affect so many other people. I thought that I was in love and I trusted the wrong people. I made money the focus of my life. I loved to have sex with the wrong people for the wrong reasons, and married the wrong men for the wrong reasons. I was lonely and desperate for a man's attention instead of being patient, virtuous, and mindful of God. I'd thought that only *other* people made those kinds of mistakes and got this disease from being gay, nasty, or stupid. I just never thought that it could ever happen to me.

But, it did --- and it can happen to you, too.

When you make a mistake, don't look back at it long.

Take the reason of the thing into your mind

and then look forward.

Mistakes are lessons of wisdom.

The past cannot be changed.

The future is yet in your power.

Hugh White (1773 - 1840)

NIAID is a component of the National Institutes of Health (NIH). NIAID supports basic and applied research to prevent, diagnose, and treat infectious and immune-mediated illnesses, including HIV/AIDS and other sexually transmitted diseases, illness from potential agents of bioterrorism, tuberculosis, malaria, autoimmune disorders, asthma and allergies.

Originally Prepared by: The Office of Communications and Public Liaison, National Institute of Allergy and Infectious Diseases National Institutes of Health, Bethesda, MD 20892

Public Health Service, U.S. Department of Health and Human Services.

Women, Children and HIV/AIDS Today HIV is
infecting a large portion of our minorities, females
and children. This section will be devoted to sites of
interest to these individuals.

HIV/AIDS Websites: Here are some interesting
websites for those who want as much information
about HIV/AIDS as they can get. These sites will be
updated as I find new ones.

- **"it"--- A Wife's Story
  <http://ourworld.compuserve.com/homepag
  es/jlamede/itpage.htm>** This site is about a
  wife's struggle in dealing with AIDS, how to
  order the book is listed here. "And so I now set
  out to tell my husband's story. There is little
  comfort in it but I hope it may, in some way,
  help others who are suffering similar torments
  to know that they are not alone. Certainly there
  is much for health workers and care providers to
  learn - so many mistakes made amongst all the
  good intentions . . ."

- **Women and HIV/AIDS Internet Resources
  <http://www.4woman.org/owh/pub/hiv-
  aids/internet.htm>** The National Women's
  Health Information Center has created this site
  just for women with HIV/AIDS. This section

lists selected World Wide Web sites on the Internet that provide information about women and HIV/AIDS. **HIV/AIDS Agencies** A selection of agencies around the United States whose primary focus is supporting, assisting and providing resources for those living with HIV and AIDS.

- **AIDS.ORG - Quality HIV/AIDS Treatment Information & Resources** **<http://www.aids.org/immunet/home.nsf/pa ge/homepage>** AIDS.Org is a great site. They list hotlines, testing sites, and other useful information, including providing updates about HIV/AIDS.

- **East Alabama AIDS Outreach** **<http://www.mindspring.net/%7Elcao/>** This website is designed to give clear facts and information about the HIV and AIDS epidemic, and what you can possibly do to help stop it. On this site are sections for news, information, volunteer information, an online support group, and links about HIV and AIDS.

- **Gay Men's Health Crisis** **<http://www.gmhc.org/>** Although the name is Gay Men's, they have programs for all populations, not just gay. I'm sure most of you know that the gay population was the hardest affected and they are the ones the created most of the support programs in use today.

- **Minnesota AIDS Project** **<http://www.mnaidsproject.org/>** MAP leads the fight against HIV and AIDS in Minnesota. Founded by a small group of dedicated volunteers in 1983, MAP has grown to a staff of more than 60 and a volunteer base of more than 1,400 to meet the challenges of this epidemic through compassionate services, prevention education and persistent advocacy on the local, state and national levels.

- **Nancy's House** **<http://nancyshouse.home.mindspring.com/ >** Nancy's House is a not-for-profit agency serving people affected or infected by HIV and AIDS in Tennessee's Bradley, Polk and McMinn counties.

- **National Native American AIDS Prevention Center** **<http://www.nnaapc.org/>** A site dedicated for the Native Americans. This is an excellent site that provides great resources and information for Native Americans.

- **Northwest AIDS Foundation**
<http://www.nwaids.org/> The Northwest AIDS Agency is one of the best agencies on the West coast. They are very involved in the Seattle area. Their website provides a host of information, resources, and help. If you're in the Seattle area and need assistance with HIV/AIDS, this is the place to check out.

- **Oak Lawn Community Services**
<http://www.olcs.org/> Oak Lawn Community Services is a progressive, not for profit organization that provides a continuum of physical and mental health services. We specialize in, but are not limited to, supporting the needs of gay men, lesbians and their families. We nurture wellness and healing for our clients. We dignify and enhance the quality of life within our community.

- **Santa Fe Cares**
<http://www.santafecares.org/> Founded in 1991, Santa Fe Cares is a community AIDS foundation providing funding for HIV/AIDS services in northern New Mexico.

- **University of Michigan HIV/AIDS Treatment Program** <http://www.med.umich.edu/hivaids/> For most Michigan residents.

- **Long Island Association for AIDS Care** <http://www.liaac.org/> LIAAC, the Long Island Association for AIDS Care, Inc., is a 501 (c) (3) not- for- profit agency that provides current information, screened referrals, educational programs and direct services to Long Island, NY residents who are concerned about HIV/AIDS.

- **Midwest AIDS Prevention Project** <http://www.aidsprevention.org/> The Midwest AIDS Prevention Project (MAPP) is one of Michigan's largest and oldest non-profit, community-based organizations whose mission is the prevention of HIV transmission through AIDS education and safer sex information. Working closely with the Michigan Department of Community Health, city and county health departments, community-based organizations and health care professionals, MAPP has developed innovative and effective behavior-based workshops, outreach projects and education programs for a wide variety of targeted populations and locations.

- **Tarrant County Fort Worth Lesbian Gay Alliance Inc. <http://pw1.netcom.com/ %7Eropertex/tclga.html>** This organization provides support to all, not just gays and lesbians, in the Fort Worth, Tarrant County of Texas.

- **HIV Insight <http://hivinsite.ucsf.edu/>** UCSF's HIV site provides informative and educational information about HIV and AIDS through a medical eye. Information is available in Spanish also. Great site!

- **The Body.com <http://www.thebody.com/index.shtml>** This is a GREAT site! It features chat, message boards, forums, facts, and more. This site provides some great information and resources as links for those living with HIV/AIDS.

- **AIDS Info NYC <http://aidsinfonyc.org/>** Providing information about medical aspects, links to educational sites and resources for those who are HIV positive, their caregivers, medical providers, friends and family.

- **Association of Nurses in AIDS Care**
  <http://www.anacnet.org/> The Association of
  Nurses in AIDS Care is a nonprofit professional
  nursing organization committed to fostering the
  individual and collective professional
  development of nurses involved in the delivery of
  health care to persons infected or affected by the
  Human Immunodeficiency Virus (HIV) and to
  promoting the health, welfare, and rights of all
  HIV infected persons.

- **John Hopkins AIDS Services**
  <http://www.hopkins-aids.edu/>
  This site continues their report by providing
  information on medicines, treatments and
  updates. Check it out!

- **NPIN Conference Calendar Database**
  <http://www.cdcnpin.org/db/public/ccmain.
  htm> This database contains information about
  conferences, seminars, and many other
  gatherings of professionals working in
  HIV/AIDS, STD, and TB prevention, treatment,
  and support services.

-

HIV/AIDS Program Index Page
<http://www.metrokc.gov/health/apu/>

If you live in Florida, then here are some resources for you to look into.

- **Mark's AIDS at About.com <http://aids.about.com/>** Mark is the guide for this site and provides some great resources and articles also.

- **The Journal of Infectious Diseases <http://www.journals.uchicago.edu/JID/journal/contents/v180n3.html>** Journals for the medical professionals to review and learn about new treatments, medications and other useful information.

Government Resources

Here is a listing of government resources concerning information, assistance, funding, and other issues related to HIV/AIDS.

- **Centers for Disease Control and Prevention <http://www.cdc.gov/nchstp/hiv_aids/dhap. htm>** This government site provides some great information on the topic of HIV/AIDS from the governmental view point. This is a great resource for all types of information.

- **National Institute of Allergy and Infectious Diseases <http://www.niaid.nih.gov/default.htm>** The NIAID provides resources on research, information, and clinical trials. If you are interested in participating in clinical trials, please search their database.

- **U.S. Food and Drug Administration <http://www.fda.gov/oashi/aids/art.html>** This is a hypertext list of FDA related HIV/AIDS articles and brochures. It's a place to find information. **News Groups** A selection of newsgroups related to HIV/AIDS.

-

* Health Boards.com**<http://www.healthboards.com/hiv-aids/>** Are you interested in becoming part of an information board about HIV/AIDS issues, if so, check out this site. They will send you information about comments and issues as submitted by various individuals.

- **PozLink - PI Treatment Mailing List <http://www.pozlink.com/>** PI-TREAT is an internet discussion list for the discussion of Protease Inhibitors and their use as treatment for HIV/AIDS. It is intended for people who are taking, anticipate taking or are interested in any way about protease inhibitors as they relate to the treatment of HIV and AIDS. **Articles & News Stories** Found on the web, these articles and news stories are of great interest.

- **AIDS Education Global Information System (AEGIS) <http://www.aegis.com/>** If you want up -to-the-minute information on news articles, press releases, government statements, and other such items, then check out this site and search until you can't type any more. There's so much on this wonderful site, that you might spend all day reading, but some of us have all day.

- **CDC's Workplace and HIV/AIDS issues**

<http://www.brta-lrta.org/> The Centers for Disease Control and Prevention Business Responds to AIDS and Labor Responds to AIDS Programs (BRTA/LRTA) help large and small businesses and labor unions meet the challenges of HIV/AIDS in the workplace and the community.

- **HIV Living: Resources for a positive life <http://www.hivliving.org/columns/>** Information, columns, HIV Dictionary, Treatments and more await those who venture here. Check it out!

- **Love & Action Ministry - caring for men, women, and children, <http://www.loveandaction.org/>** Providing a spritual resources for all people living with HIV/AIDS, their friends, family and caregivers.

- **Tucson Interfaith HIV/AIDS Network <http://www.tihan.org/>** The Tucson Interfaith HIV/AIDS Network, through the efforts of many volunteers, ensures accurate information regarding HIV and AIDS is available to all of our communities in Tucson.

- **The HIV/AIDS Ministries Network - United Methodist Church <http://gbgm-umc.org/programs/hiv/aids.html>** The United Methodist Church has created a christian based program with information, assistance, and most importantly love for those with HIV/AIDS.

A quick note about the King of Swaziland, Mswati III.

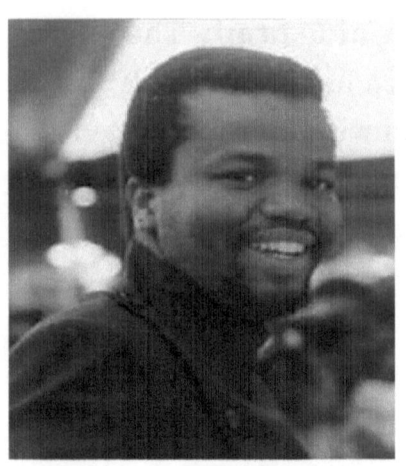 My apologies for the reference to his country in my story. This manuscript was written in 2006, and honestly, I knew very little about King Mswati or Swaziland, except that he was one of the most good-looking African men I had ever seen in my life, and his country is suffering tremendously under the stigma of a high incidence of HIV/AIDS cases. The king has 13 wives and 27 children. He is also under a lot of stress and political pressure in the current administration of Swaziland's Republic. Apparently, his sexual prowess is legendary as the following news article confirms.

Swazi queens revolt - 04/07/2004 08:38-(SA)

Sikhumbuzo Ndiweni

Johannesburg -

Palace revolt by Swazi queens allegedly over concerns about contracting Aids has resulted in two of them fleeing Swaziland, with more believed to follow suit. Queen Putsoana Hwale left Swaziland on June 24 with a coterie of bodyguards and was on Saturday in Protea

Glen, Soweto. It is believed that King Mswati ordered her to leave the palace.

According to royal sources, Queen Delisa Magwaza, popularly known as La Magwaza, had left the palace two weeks before and is now in London. La Magwaza was last year embroiled in a highly publicized affair with a Soweto man, Lizo Shabangu, who spilled the beans when she told him she was ending the affair. Shabangu at the time said La Magwaza had told him she was starved for attention and love as Mswati often didn't visit her for months on end. This caused tension in her relationship with the king.

It is understood that the root of the problem is the continuous annual inflow of young girls being added to Mswati's list of wives. Some of the young girls are believed to have had boyfriends before marrying the king. The queens felt this exposed them to the dangers of contracting diseases such as HIV/Aids. The king recently married Zena Mahlangu, 19, his 11th wife.

This caused anger among the other wives because she had had a highly publicized affair before being picked to be yet another queen. Mswati has also taken Nomonde Fihla, 18, who now lives in one of the palaces, as a queen in waiting. She is a former Miss Swaziland. The king's alleged extra-marital affairs have caused great unhappiness among his wives.

Sources in Swaziland said Mswati visited Hwale after La Magwaza's departure, and found that her bags were packed and she was getting ready to leave.

He apparently ordered three elders and 10 bodyguards (six of whom are women) to accompany her to Soweto. A close relative led a City Press team to La Hwale's father's house in Protea Glen where a tri-nation meeting was in progress between Hwale's relatives from Lesotho, where her parents live, the Swazi contingent and her South African relatives.

Several cars with Swaziland government number plates were parked outside with guards posted around the area. A relative of Hwale's, from Alexandra, told City Press that the family had been mediating with the Swazi royal house for the past five months over Hwale's dissatisfaction. He said Hwale's appearance in Soweto had been a surprise to the family.

Mswati, 36, has decreed that girls should not engage in pre-marital sex, and girls in Swaziland wear a ribbon to indicate their "purity".

He has, however, not strictly adhered to his own principles. Mswati is believed to have recently forced Marwick Khumalo, a speaker in parliament, to resign due to his alleged affair with one of the older queens.

Author's Biography:

C.J. Green is a former actor, singer, model, and dancer who grew up on Long Island in New York. She attended college and graduated with a B.S. degree in Business Administration, but a too early marriage, quick divorce and pregnancy prevented her from pursuing her business career to its fullest. After several attempts to obtain a Master's Degree; being thwarted by bad relationships, custody battles, and severe financial hardships caused by physical illness, (at one point she was home-less for several months in Atlanta, GA and in Las Vegas, NV) she turned to writing for therapy. She also had a short, but successful career designing clothing and novelties while writing and editing manuscripts for others in her spare time.

Writing has always been one of her greatest passions and she dreamed of publishing books about the challenges that young adults face in the Age of Sexual Revolution to help people understand how difficult the job of "parent" has become in this century.

"Our world has changed so tremendously in the fifty years since the "Happy Days" and "Father Knows Best" parenting of the sixties, " she says.

"The innocence of childhood has been totally destroyed and replaced with the unbridled, uncontrolled passions and anger of youth gone wild."

Parents have got to regain control of their children before it's too late.

Hopefully, she prays this book will help.